SOUP CLEANSE
cookbook

SOUP CLEANSE

cookbook

EMBRACE A BETTER BODY AND A HEALTHIER YOU WITH THE WEEKLY SOUP PLAN

NICOLE CENTENO

founder of
SPLENDID
SPOON

RODALE

RODALE *wellness*

Live happy. Be healthy. Get inspired.

Sign up today to get exclusive access to our authors, exclusive bonuses,
and the most authoritative, useful, and cutting-edge information on health, wellness,
fitness, and living your life to the fullest.

Visit us online at RodaleWellness.com
Join us at RodaleWellness.com/Join

Rodale books may be purchased for business or promotional use or for special sales.
For information, please write to:
Special Markets Department, Rodale Inc., 733 Third Avenue, New York, NY 10017

Printed in the United States of America

Rodale Inc. makes every effort to use acid-free ♾, recycled paper ♲.

Photographs by Tara Donne

Book design by Christina Gaugler

Library of Congress Cataloging-in-Publication Data is on file with the publisher.

ISBN 978–1–62336–731–2

Distributed to the trade by Macmillan

2 4 6 8 10 9 7 5 3 1 paperback

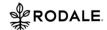

We inspire health, healing, happiness, and love in the world.
Starting with you.

For Mom

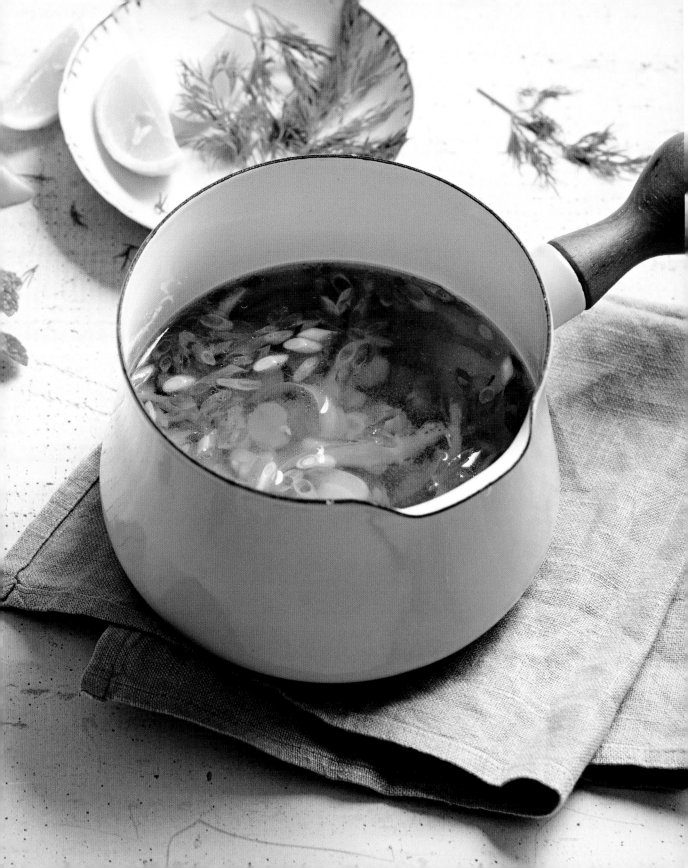

CONTENTS

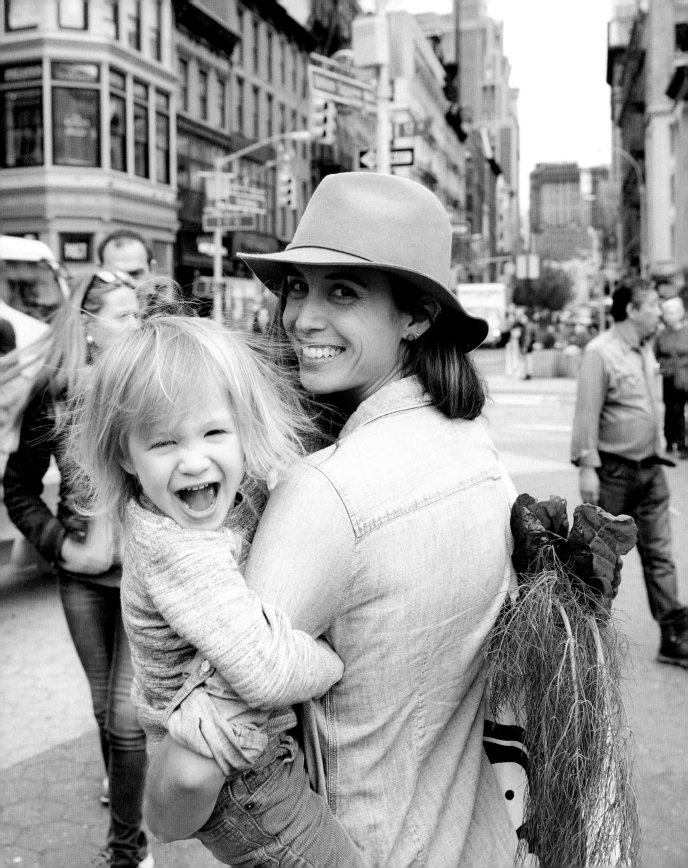

INTRODUCTION

"HOBIE, PLEASE STOP BARKING," I pleaded. The buzzer of my Brooklyn apartment wailed, and my high-anxiety dog was not having it. My 2-month-old was wailing, too; he had just barfed two boobs' worth of breast milk all over himself and me. Is something wrong with him? I wondered as I struggled to hold my crying baby, turn on the bath, and remove my milk-soaked pants. And then Hobie, likely because of his high anxiety, barfed, too. I walked, one yoga-pant-leg-on-one-leg-off, like a *Walking Dead* extra to the kitchen and grabbed a dish towel. Up until this very moment I stood firmly in the no-paper-towel camp. Waste paper when I could use a reusable towel? Nonsense! A more realistic version of my self seemed to be giggling from the sidelines: I'll show you nonsense. I made a mental note to keep paper towels in stock. I could feel the sweat prickling the back of my neck, the knots in my shoulders hot with stress and the weight of my newborn. The tears would be next. This is survival mode now. Get it together, I told myself.

Just one leg in front of the other and focus on bathing yourself and your baby. It's not so bad! Barf is not the end of the world! Drop a towel on the dog barf, handle baby barf first. Undress baby. Phone rings. Naked baby continues to protest. It's my kitchen production manager; I must answer the phone. "Hello?" Drape baby in a towel so he doesn't succumb to hypothermia. "I'm so sorry. That's Grover crying. What's up?" I ask. "What?!

The soup is what temperature?" Someone had left the door open to the refrigerated space where my soup was being stored before its delivery to my biggest-very-big-deal account. In the sweltering July heat, the soup had risen to 70 degrees. It was spoiled, for those of you less familiar with the rules of safe food storage. The tears came. The buzzer screamed again. It's my mom. Oh, it's my *mom* who is buzzing. Thank God I asked her to come over. How could I have forgotten?

And that was the day over a thousand pounds of asparagus soup went bad. A short 24 hours earlier, over 2,000 pounds of locally sourced asparagus had arrived from a family-owned farm in Long Island (in hand-stamped wooden crates, no less). The crisp green spears had been trimmed by hand then blanched and dunked into an ice bath before meeting their soupy fate. My crew of two had made asparagus stock with the woody asparagus stems to ensure we pulled every last nutrient and flavor molecule out and into the soup. A crate of lemons had been zested and squeezed by hand. The pulpy citrus juice had been added a little at a time to balance the green flavor of the asparagus, the brininess of sea salt, and the richness of the olive oil. It was a vibrant life-giving green puree that was satisfying and refreshing all at once. And now this crew of two was opening every hand-labeled container and dumping it down the drain. If I was to save face with my big-deal customer, I needed to figure out a way to remake the entire batch that was due to them in a few hours.

Life grows full very quickly. In 4 short years, I have gone to culinary school, launched a business, had my first baby, managed an evolving business, had my second beautiful baby, and embraced the changing dynamic of a growing family. And yet, I have a growing list of things I want to do even more of: more reading, more running, more meditating, more concertgoing, more time with my friends—more baths! I have noticed a similar phenomenon with my girlfriends and Splendid Spoon clients. We are saying yes more often. Yes to work. Yes to family. Yes to eating well. Yes to all the elements that excite our senses, feed our curiosity, and stimulate a deeper engagement with the world. It's possible, but we sometimes forget that simplicity is paramount.

Before I launched Splendid Spoon, I had a laughably naive perspective on what it meant to simplify:

I drew Venn diagrams. I thought if I could find the place where all my yeses intersected, I would have the key! Like a linchpin for my perfectly organized, highly productive life, that center of the Venn would be my answer. It looked like the drawing below.

The sheer stupidity of this Venn diagram is embarrassing to the point of being hilarious now. I mean, starting a business was my answer? Take it from my milk- and soup-drenched yoga pants, my friends, if simplicity is the most important lesson of all, then you have to go one step at a time.

There were many heart swells and heartbreaks as I attempted to tackle and ultimately abandon this Venn diagram philosophy. The asparagus soup saga revealed that I hadn't found my linchpin; I had burnt a whole through the center of my neat little Venn diagram. My eyelashes weren't just singed; my hair was on fire. We all do it. We have

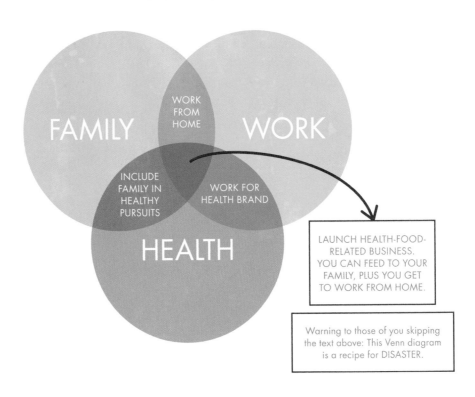

a tendency to get excited about projects and relationships and to work hard on those things, often prioritizing them over our own needs. It was like I had gotten so excited about my new roles as mom and CEO that I had left a critical part of me behind: the part of me that stands up for what I need. It's the part of me that believes yoga and meditation are just as important as the weekly team meeting. It's the part of me that says, Slow down, you'll make better decisions if you get a full night's rest. I wanted to be a kick-ass mom and a successful business leader, but I had forgotten that being great for other people meant being great to Nicole first.

So I tossed my old Venn diagram in the trash and embraced a simplified version of saying yes. Instead of overlapping all my wishes and dreams to form a diagram of how to support everything at once, I said yes to myself first. I channeled a future version of myself who said, You deserve this, Nicole! You are a strong, smart, and driven woman. You deserve to spend more time on you so you can accomplish your goals, and enjoy the journey you are on! Saying yes to me was critical, but getting to that future version of myself took a little more planning. It's one thing to identify where you want to go, and it's another to actually get there.

I wrote down words that described my future self: *healthy, energized, productive, joyful,* and *engaged*. These were my intentions, and the first word said a lot: *healthy*. Taking care of my health was first and foremost. You are what you eat, after all. When I went full time as an entrepreneur and launched Splendid Spoon in early 2013, it was with the intention to increase my veggie intake during my first pregnancy. I had focused on developing lots of plant-based soups because eating mostly vegan made me feel really great during and shortly after my pregnancy. What I hadn't done was create a plan around those soups, and a plan was what I needed. It was time to rewire my habits to support my growing life. The Soup Cleanse was born.

I had all the tools to put together a simplified approach to my well-being: I had studied metabolism and the benefits of ancient diet therapies like fasting, I was a trained chef, and I knew from experience that meditation and mindfulness would keep me more committed to my plan so I could reach my goals. My background gave me the unique advantage of being able to put this approach together quickly and effectively, and it worked. I can say with confidence that I am healthy, energized, productive, incredibly joyful, and engaged in my life. It's not always perfect, but I have found a sense of equilibrium, and it has everything to do with my Soup Cleanse program. Now, I can share it with you so you too can stand up straight, look yourself in the mirror, and say yes.

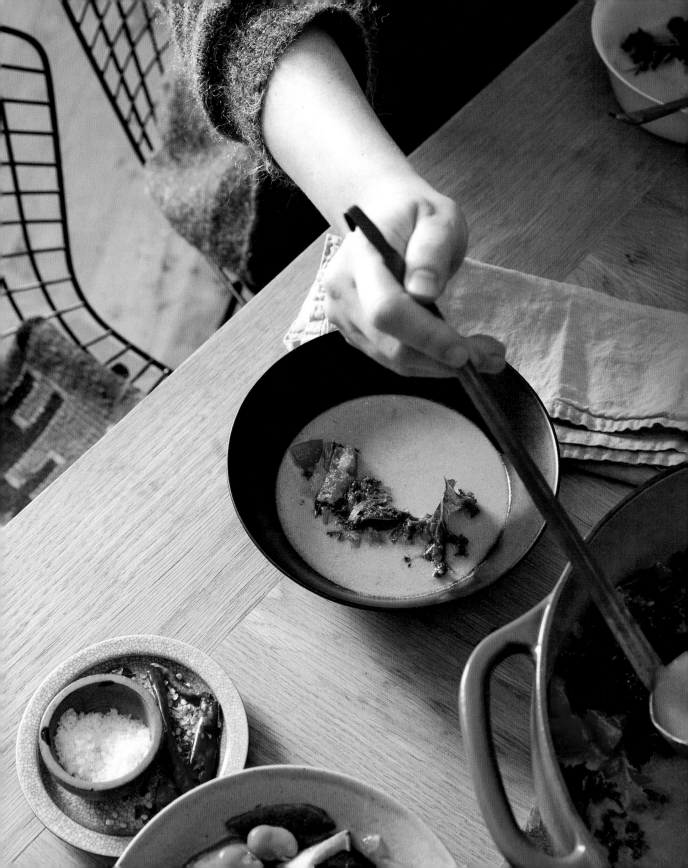

part 1

THE
SOUP
BASICS

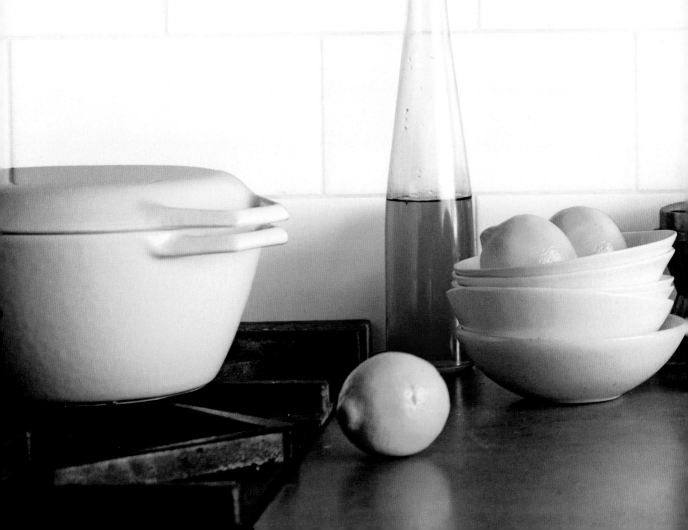

chapter 1

ANOTHER CLEANSE?!

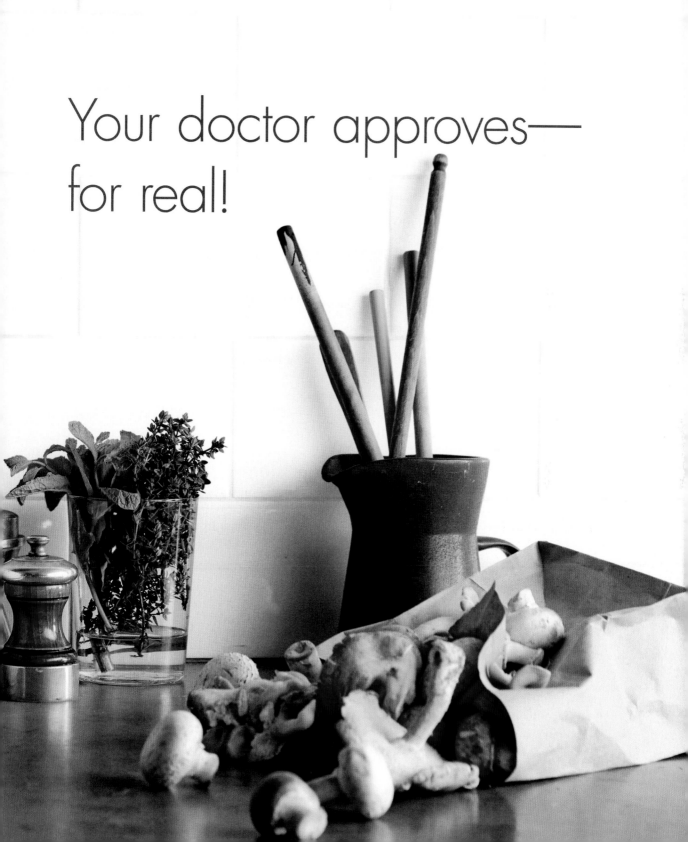

Your doctor approves—
for real!

A CLEANSE? REALLY? THAT'S THE ANSWER?

The last thing a driven, productive person needs is a complicated diet that creates more work and causes anxiety. Often, the simplest answer is the right one, and that's the case with the Soup Cleanse. Unlike other so-called cleanses, my Soup Cleanse isn't a quick fix. It's a regular routine that combines a higher-intensity reset along with my simple meal swaps to maintain great health while allowing lots of flexibility to (gasp!) eat things other than soup. The Soup Cleanse is based on the principle that small changes made every day produce big results.

It's true: Our bodies have wonderful natural cleansing mechanisms. The liver removes toxins from our blood, and the kidneys further filter that blood and make sure those toxins are excreted properly. When I talk about a soup cleanse, I mean this to be an opportunity to help your organs do the good job they already do; to provide your cells with exclusively plant-based fuel; and to increase your absorption of antioxidants, which help combat diseases and improve the function of your circulatory, cardiovascular, and digestive systems. There is loads of research that shows just how much better our bodies run when we give them more plant-based nutrients.

Eating more plants and eating primarily because you're hungry (also known as portion control) are key components of any healthy lifestyle. But we often fail at this because of our environment; temptations, triggers, and old habits throw us off course and keep us in a frustrating cycle of knowing what we want but not sticking to an action plan. Creating new patterns that are healthier than current patterns is the key, but change is tough. We create new patterns and stick to them when we receive a reward (the quicker we receive the reward, the bet-

ter) and when the new patterns are actually simpler than the old ones (like texting with a friend instead of using voice calls and voicemail). This is the essence of the Soup Cleanse. I wanted to create new patterns that made me feel so good that I would stick with them forever. When we get a reward from a simpler pattern, then everything makes sense. I call this practicality.

Soup is the perfect food for creating new patterns because many of us have positive emotional connections to soup—a loved one serving us a bowl after playing in the snow all day, cozying up to a big bowl on a sick day, making a pot of chili with friends for a tailgate party. Soup unifies, soup heals, and soup makes us feel good. It's also perfect for all sorts of science-y reasons. Soup keeps you satisfied with a lower caloric density, and because it is usually cooked, the digestive process starts before you have your first spoonful, meaning your body can absorb and use the nutrients more readily. These were the main reasons I started cooking soup.

Before I launched Splendid Spoon, I had another soup company: Sea Bean Goods. This was a pop-up and catering project I embarked on while I continued to work full-time in advertising at Condé Nast. For 2½ years I souped on the side to test my chops as a professional cook and entrepreneur. Around 4 a.m. I would splash cold water on my face, hop on my bike, and ride to a pizza kitchen on Greenpoint Avenue in Brooklyn. If you had one of my soups from 2011 to 2012, there is a good chance it was made in a small pot next to a screaming-hot brick pizza oven. Working next to that oven before an 8-hour day at the office tested my mettle, but my physical fatigue inspired some of Splendid Spoon's bestselling flavors. Soup became my solace, my energy, and my fortitude. Above all, it became my go-to meal when I was dog-tired at various points during those 15-hour days. I'd sip soup on ice in the morning, pour it into thermoses for a hot lunch, and savor a bowl for dinner. I'd always share with my colleagues and friends. There were many days when all I ate was soup.

Eating soup simplified my life in this way. Truthfully, I would have been eating croissants all day if I had been a croissant maker. But (thankfully) there was a healthful reward with eating soup that kept me going back for more. Actually, there were three rewards: (1) It was convenient to eat any time, hot or cold. (2) It was satisfying for several hours. (3) I had more energy and was even opting for more vegetable-centric food when I cooked nonsoup meals. These were all positive things, but I knew that in order for eating soup to really become a lasting pattern, I would need to up the ante in the rewards department.

Meditation and mindfulness have been a positive part of my life since I first studied Buddhism as a young child. I remember staring intently at a sculpture of the Buddha at RISD (Rhode Island School of Design). His expression was placid, content. He was so comforting to look at that I found myself gazing at him long after the group had moved on. I continued my own research into meditation (or mindfulness, as it's often referred to in Buddhism and as I'll refer to it in this book) and its effects on the body and mind. Was this really the key to peace and happiness? Maybe. But more importantly for souping, there's an immediate reward with mindfulness.

Taking your time when you eat is a form of mindfulness. Your mind is nudged into a connection with your body's actions because you eat soup more slowly than you eat a sandwich, drink a smoothie, or twirl up forkfuls of pasta. Yes, you can slow down your eating of any food or beverage, but soup really helps you slow down because it's often warm (pause, blow, sip tentatively) and because it's liquid (fill the spoon, not too much, that's just right, now lift carefully lest you dribble that broth down your chin). When we take a few extra minutes to connect our minds to our bodies through mindfulness, we create positive new connections in our brains. We stimulate endorphins. We settle the mind and unlock its reward center. Practicing mindfulness regularly and over time is proven to have really profound effects on our health and happiness, and many of us gain a sense of calm and clarity even after only 5 to 10 minutes of mindful exercise.

My weekly souping plan wraps four very powerful elements together: plant-based nutrition, practicality, portion control (intermittent fasting), and mindfulness. I call these the four pillars, and they support the foundation for a better me, a better you, a more Splendid Self. (I describe these in more detail below.) The idea is that the soup does a lot of the heavy lifting for you by pulling these four elements together. All you have to do is invite those soup rituals into your weekly routine.

Still unsure of this whole doctor-approved thing? You will be hard-pressed to find a physician who does not agree with my philosophy: Eat more vegetables, practice portion control, and embrace small changes that can become long-lasting habits. These behaviors are paramount to creating a healthier relationship with food. There are no quick fixes, but sometimes the most nourishing, simple solutions can truly enhance your life. That's how souping works. It's not a quick fix, but it is simple, and it will enhance your life. Bring this book to your next doctor's visit, and ask her if she agrees.

Arts and Sciences

My grandfather was a surgeon, his sister was a pediatric specialist, my aunt is an allergist, and my uncle is also a practicing physician. Growing up with doctors in my family meant looking at the human body as a set of intricate systems—so if you're sick, it means one of those systems needs fixing. I have always respected the scientific process for explaining how things work and for offering solutions to what ails us. But while my dad's side of the family was governed by the rules of Western medicine, my mom's side of the family embraced the power of Mother Nature to alleviate and prevent ailments. To this day, when I have a cold, my dad will offer a decongestant and my mom will make me a scalding hot tea of echinacea, goldenrod, and licorice and prescribe a day of rest.

My mom—while respectful of the need for traditional medicine in extreme circumstances—believes that 99 percent of our ailments are not extreme. She taught me that most of what ails us can be alleviated or prevented by eating more vegetables, moving more, and laughing a lot. Get fresh air every day. Embrace the people you love. Dive into the ocean whenever possible. And the various things that push our limits of patience and tolerance every day—don't analyze them so much. The saying "Don't sweat the small stuff" was uttered frequently in my childhood home. Stress less and let go more. I always loved the positive reinforcement of my mom's approach to health. It felt more like an art than a science to place faith in my body and trust its ability to strengthen and support me. However, I am my father's daughter, and I enjoy the confidence of knowing my wellness choices are backed by science.

The point is, science is important, but it's not all or nothing. We are fortunate to live during a time when people can dedicate their lives to scientific research that helps us understand how to live longer, happier lives. Practically speaking, though, most of us don't want to agonize over the relative health benefits of broccoli versus spinach. It's not a comfortable existence to require scientific proof for every choice you make, especially when you're hungry for dinner.

It's great, for example, to plan out a week of healthy, plant-based meals but counterproductive to get stressed when a good friend throws a last-minute birthday party smack in the middle of your week. Instead of thinking about the party as a collision with your best-laid plans, maybe embrace the fact that socializing with your buddies will have a positive impact on your well-being, too—and have a bowl of soup before the party so you go for a smaller slice of cake. Life is full of surprises and gray areas and unpredictability, so why should our approach to health be all or nothing? Stressing about the last-minute changes to your daily life will only serve to erode your feelings of confidence. Souping is about acknowledging that we do the best we can to make healthy choices, that our bodies benefit from all sorts of small changes, and that having confidence in ourselves is absolutely the best feeling of all.

I created the Soup Cleanse so I didn't have to agonize about my food choices. Everyone talks about balance, but it feels a lot more like juggling. Before we can balance all the meaningful elements that make up a life, it's important to strengthen what's inside us first. Think of it like this: You don't go into a full headstand when you walk into a yoga class; first you find your center through breathing and core-strengthening poses to support the more challenging ones. I created the weekly Soup Cleanse Plan out of an unavoidable need to center myself. It started with a big dose of self-love so I could build from the inside out.

This all may sound like common sense, but it really took some time for me to fully grasp just how important it was to prioritize my own health. I had been selling soup and working on recipes for over a year as a side gig to my full-time job in media strategy at Condé Nast, but it wasn't until I became pregnant that Splendid Spoon launched as a plant-based wellness brand, and it wasn't until the great asparagus fiasco of 2013 that the 7-day plan was born as a remedy to my demanding life.

This book is the culmination of many fits and starts and failed attempts, spilled soup, spoiled soup, exploding soup, and botched flavors. I've simplified and distilled all my lessons into an incredibly easy plan that anyone can follow and anyone with any dietary preferences can adapt for improved health. The plan is driven by my (and now Splendid Spoon's) four-pillar philosophy: plant-based nutrition, practicality, portion control (intermittent fasting), and mindfulness. Soup helps me be the best I can be because it is rooted in a foundation that supports me rather than asking me to do more. Here is the story of how these pillars came to be.

Grown Woman Seeking Plant-Based Nutrition:
My Less-Than-Splendid Former Self

The average American's diet is 28 percent animal products, 41 percent fatty and sugary "extras," 23 percent grains, and only 8 percent fruits and vegetables.[1, 2] Sixty-nine percent of us are overweight.[3] And the leading causes of death are heart disease, cancer, and lower respiratory diseases.[4] There is no doubt that eating a diet rich in vegetables improves health in a multitude of ways, from decreasing the likelihood of type 2 diabetes and many cancers to improving life span and literally every system in our bodies.[5] Yet, 87 percent of Americans don't eat enough vegetables.[6] This is not right. Something is awry. What's wrong here?

Avoiding vegetables is, unfortunately, the path of least resistance. This reality really bugs me because I know (and so do you) how great vegetables are for health. The uphill battle to get more veggies into our diets is due in no small part to what's available at restaurants and as packaged convenience food. It's also due to the fact that rich,

sugary, starchy, salty food sets off all sorts of pleasure signals in our brains, and it creates a bit of an addiction to those things.

My own diet was evidence of this and hit its apex while I was in school at The French Culinary Institute in Manhattan in 2010. I consumed an excessive amount of meat. And potatoes had "somehow" become my go-to vegetable of choice—thanks, culinary school, for the 101 ways to mash, fry, and sauté spuds. I went through about a pound of butter a week because it had crept into literally every recipe I concocted. I frequently managed to subvert the amazing health benefits of spinach, for example, by smothering it in roux and drowning it in cream and cheese. I was driven by taste and only taste.

The idea of making food that was good for me had become an afterthought. Yes, it's important to make food that tickles your taste buds in all the right ways, but I felt completely off balance. Food was like a drug. Consuming intensely fatty, sugary, and salty food is satisfying and enjoyable for the duration of the meal, but I crashed shortly after eating and also in almost every other aspect of my life. I needed a steady stream of caffeine throughout the day to feel normal at work, I classified granola bars as a food group, I let off steam at the end of the day with a huge glass (or three, let's be real) of red wine, and I kept my weight in check by running or spinning like a woman on the verge of a nervous breakdown.

When I got pregnant in late 2012, the reality of my diet came crashing in on me. How had this happened? I had studied biology in college, focusing on diet therapies, of all things. I was ashamed, honestly, because I couldn't cry ignorance. I knew from the work I had done in the research lab that what you eat has an incredibly powerful effect on your well-being, and yet I had a quart of duck fat in my fridge. And honestly (and possibly TMI), I did not poop every day back then. It's weird how that really affects you in a negative way. It can be distracting sitting there with all that compacted meat and potatoes in your lower intestines. You just don't feel right. I remember sitting on the toilet one day thinking, This is why Mom tells us to eat our roughage; I need to eat more vegetables. I imagined my baby not growing big enough as he struggled to suck nutrients out of a steady stream of marbled steak and peanut butter soufflé. I was hopeful that I could quickly propel myself into a cleaner way of living, but what I really needed was food rehab.

Surprise, surprise—going cold turkey isn't so easy in our world of catered pizza lunches, artisan-pastry-laden cafés, and Doritos at the checkout. The majority of food companies out there are churning out very convenient, nutrient-deficient foods. It's estimated that 61 percent of our calories come from highly processed food.[7] And that highly processed food served a purpose, as evidenced by my penchant for granola bars (convenience rules in the life of a modern woman). This was my conundrum as I approached clean eating. Why was it so inconvenient to make a simple shift that would definitely improve my health? Why was it so hard to get my veggies?

I created a "yes" list (whole grains, cooked and raw vegetables, nuts, whole fruit) and a "never" list (takeout, anything with more than 8 grams of sugar in a serving, premade snacks, anything sold in crinkly bags). I bought copious amounts of fresh vegetables at the farmers' market and pledged to cook all my meals. This was a fail. Inevitably, I would cave in and opt for takeout after a 12-hour day. I would guzzle a sugar-loaded yogurt smoothie during a 3 p.m. slump. I'd bargain with myself at social gatherings: If I skip the buffalo wings, I can have a pint of IPA—shoot, how many grams of sugar are in the IPA? Many beets and carrots withered in the wake of this failed solution, and worse, every misstep made me feel like a loser.

I tried expensive meal-delivery services, with my frustration reaching fever pitch at lunchtime as I realized my $17 salad was wilting in the fridge at home. I pondered juicing. Did it make sense to concentrate a basket's worth of produce into a single glass of juice, essentially a very expensive sugary beverage? Probably not, my rational self answered. But all those lovely models sipping green juice couldn't be wrong, right? Going against all sense of reason, I dove headlong into a ginger-spiked pool of kale, cucumber, and lemon with a 3-day cleanse, thinking maybe it could be a quick fix every month. I missed chewing and failed to grasp the positive health benefit of what was effectively another highly processed food: lots of fruit juice, no fiber, and a lot of sexy marketing. I'd been had by those lovely models and their long legs and white teeth, mysteriously void of beet juice stains.

Juicing was like the visual equivalent of my fatty French cooking: beautiful to look at, easy going down, and then *crash*. Same as butter and duck fat, those pretty juices played to the pleasure principle. I did learn something really valuable from the juices and meal kits, though: They provided a simple program to follow. I hadn't found a program that worked for me, but there was something nice about having the weekly structure. Step 1, Step 2, Step 3, repeat.

At this point I had been making soup for about a year in that pizza kitchen, but I hadn't developed a formal program around souping. My diet had gotten *better* with soup, but it wasn't the best it could be because I hadn't created a foolproof (me-proof) program to stay in line. I needed a little tough love—a simple plan that allowed for flexibility, but a structured program nonetheless. It took me until after the birth of amazing baby #1 (Hi, Grover!) to come up with all the pieces that would become the 7-day plan.

Making Hard Stuff Practical for the Modern Woman

The existing healthy-eating programs just added more complexity to my life. I wanted a plan with enough structure so that even my easily distracted brain could stay focused but with enough nimbleness to accommodate my dynamic life. Nothing stays the same, after all, so why should my diet be super rigid?

Too often, diets get in the way of social engagements and make people feel like they aren't part of the gang because their diets won't allow happy hour snacks. This is usually where diets fail. The emotional pressure to feel connected to friends and family through food can be intense, and without good habits to support you, it can be near impossible to stay on track.

I started putting together the weekly Soup Cleanse Plan when I was pregnant with my first son. No, I did not restrict myself to just soup. No, I was not looking to lose weight while I was pregnant. I was absolutely looking for a structure that would help me choose my healthy soup instead of a 99-cent piece of pizza (or one of those amazing blistery crust pizzas made in a coal- or wood-fired oven, for that matter). Brooklyn really has a lot of good pizza options—but I digress. See, even as I write, it's easy for me to get distracted! The

plan made it easier to choose healthy instead of mozzarella-y. It started like this: Pick one meal a day that would be soup. Full stop. That was it. I knew that building sound habits was critical for my (and my growing family's) long-term health. The more complex the solution, the less likely I was to stick with it. I stocked my fridge with soup. And there was always a surplus, so I never got stuck.

After the birth of Grover (and after the first 2 months of pure adrenaline and amazement and fatigue and chaos that come with a newborn), I wanted to get back to my fighting weight, so to speak. My daily soup meals had kept me in great shape throughout my pregnancy, but I really wanted to discard my maternity pants. No matter what your body type, there's something symbolic about throwing out the stretch pants you wear well past your baby's birth. It was less about my weight and more about what it meant for me as a woman. Discarding those pants reminded me that in addition to being a new mom, I was also a fit woman, a sexy woman. Getting back to regular pants (not necessarily even prepregnancy clothes—just *not* maternity clothes) reconnected me with myself as an individual. I wasn't carrying my baby inside me anymore. The next phase of my child's life had begun, and he was his own entity. So was I.

I wanted to burn those damn maternity pants. This was when I added a full day of souping to my weekly routine. I realized that with this lean day of eating, plus the soup meal replacements on the other days of the week, I had created a system of intermittent fasting. This was interesting because I knew from my work in the research lab that there were a lot of benefits to fasting. I'll talk more about this in the next section, but note that the structure of the 7-day plan was fully formed at this point, and it was very simple: 1 Soup Cleanse Day (all soup, all day), 5 Soup Swap Days (replacing one meal a day with soup), 1 Wander Day (a day of no rules).

The plan worked because there was a ton of flexibility but also enough structure to keep me in a healthy cycle week after week for a positive cumulative impact on my health. The Wander Day enabled me to go to birthday parties and have a day of pancakes *and* beer. It felt like a reasonable and laid-back way to enjoy whatever I felt like, without feeling like a crazy day of indulgences to "reward" myself for restrictive eating. It felt natural. The Soup Swap Days brought consistency to every day without feeling restrictive or boring. The Soup Cleanse Day reliably reset my habits week after week and kept my veggie intake way up. It was a plan. It was practical. I was just about there.

So the structure of the weekly soup plan has been outlined now. Most wellness and diet books jump right into the how-to at this point. And you could totally do that: Skip ahead to "The Four Pillars of Souping" on page 14 and then to Chapter 3. It won't hurt my feelings. If, however, you really want to connect to the "why" and give yourself a much greater chance of success, read on to learn more about the science behind my weekly Soup Cleanse Plan and to see why souping is the most natural way for your body to find her balance.

There's some history ahead, and then I get a little heady by diving into the power of mindfulness. In Chapter 2, I reveal even more of the power of soup and veggies. You say you want to change your life for better—and forever? You say you want to be your most Splendid Self? Let's spoon.

The History of Intermittent Fasting

Let's take it back. Like, way back. To 100,000 years ago, when humans first went upright and started running around, becoming hunters and foragers. Back then, heart disease wasn't the leading cause of death, there wasn't an obesity epidemic, and cancers were virtually nonexistent. I'm not saying our ancient human ancestors didn't have problems; violent death rates were certainly much higher, and the leading cause of death for women was related to childbirth. The point is that most of the illnesses that plague the human race today are relatively new when you look at how long we've been roaming around on earth. The profile of our health changed dramatically with the advent of modern agriculture a short 2,000 years ago. In the past 200 years, we have streamlined agriculture so much that we have monocrops without the genetic diversity that benefits our bodies, and over a third of our calories now come from fats and sugars added to packaged foods.[8]

The most convenient foods are calorie-dense and nutrient-deficient. Big companies have poured billions of dollars into food marketing to create desire and demand for food that should be classified as a drug: high-sugar, high-salt, high-calorie products that have literally no nutritional value save the caloric energy they provide. And you know what, the pleasure principle works well in business. It feels good to eat crap—like oh-hell-yes-these-chips-are-the-shit-and-I-will-eat-this-whole-bag-because-I-cannnn—for a hot second. And then there's every other not-hot second of living your regular life. Those lame-ass seconds of I feel like shit; I wish my pants buttoned; why haven't I pooped in 3 days; I don't have time to cook and now I feel shitty about that, too, so I guess I'll go to that burrito place and pile on the queso because then I'll get to that hot second of awesome again. It's a truly vicious cycle.

In recent years, physicians and scientists have scrutinized our modern diet and how detrimental to our health it really is. And there has been a big focus on reuniting our modern selves with our ancestral health. Take a look at societies that transition to a more Western diet, and you'll see they get an extra side of Western diseases along with their Frappuccinos and chicken nuggets. Diabetes was virtually unknown, for instance, among the Maya of Central America until the 1950s, when they switched to a Western diet high in sugars and the rate of diabetes skyrocketed.[9]

The Paleo diet is probably the most popular of the diets inspired by ancestral behaviors. Paleo tells us that protein should make up 30 percent of our diets. I'm personally not paleo because I like all the great environmental impacts of eating mostly plant-based (check out the Bonus section in "The Four Pillars of Souping," page 15). That said, paleo works really well for a growing number of people, and souping can even augment this lifestyle by incorporating some lean eating into the diet. Amanda G. Henry, PhD, a paleobiologist at the Max Planck Institute for Evolutionary Anthropology

in Leipzig, Germany, has revealed that our ancestors may have craved a lot of meat but they subsisted mostly on plants, and while 30 percent of their annual calories came from animal proteins, they also "endured lean times when they [ate] less than a handful of meat each week."[10]

Humans are biologically built as hunters and foragers. Before the rise of modern agriculture, we had to hunt and kill our food, often subsisting for weeks at a time on a mostly plant-based diet. There would be lean days with less to eat and fat days with more to eat after a hunt. These lean, plant-based days were much more frequent than the fat ones. Today, communities that practice this type of mostly plant-based lifestyle with several lean days throughout the week live longer and have a much lower incidence of heart disease, diabetes, and cancer.[11] Achieving your ideal body weight is a fantastic side effect, but the goal is really to gain a sense of balance as well as a true escape from the harmful cycles of the typical American diet.

The science of souping includes the theory that fasting has many positive effects on our health. Abstaining from certain foods or from food altogether for a period of time, in an effort to purify mind and body, is an ancient therapy. Every major religion practices fasting to produce spiritual benefits. Ancient philosophers like Aristotle, Plato, and Socrates encouraged fasting for its healing properties. Ayurvedic and yogic practices, thousands of years old, include fasting for its therapeutic properties. The benefits of fasting include increased longevity, increased energy, and weight loss, and the cool thing is that you don't have to go for days without food to reap these benefits.

The soup cleanse is a form of fasting because you are abstaining from many of the other foods you might eat on a regular basis. Doctors call this intermittent fasting, and it is proven to help our bodies become more resistant to disease, to reduce inflammation, and to prevent many of the physical effects of aging.[12] Some of the research around intermittent fasting has been inspired by communities where more people live to the age of 100 and rates of cancer, heart disease, and diabetes are significantly lower than for the average American. The research around long-lived communities also reveals that members of these communities eat far less meat than we do now.[13] Of course, you don't have to be current on publications from the clinical research community to know that eating more vegetables is great for your health, and increased vegetable intake is a big part of the formula for the cleanse. You do not have to be a 100 percent vegan to benefit from the positive effects of the Soup Cleanse. The point is that the soups reduce your overall caloric intake and increase the number of plant-based meals you consume over the course of a week.

Depending on the regimen you choose, it will probably be lower in calories than you are accustomed to, and unless you are already vegan, you will be taking a break from meat and dairy. When you focus on plant-based food during key days and meals throughout the week, and week after week, you reset your metabolism to support a healthier body.

The Art of Mindfulness

The final, all-important component of the plan that needed to be addressed was habit. Over 60 percent of women gain more weight than they initially set out to lose after quitting a diet. You can't hop on and off the foundation when it works for you; you have to *be* the foundation. The key to maintaining good health is building simple behaviors that reward you so that you repeat them over and over again. Repeat enough times, and that behavior becomes a true habit.

This isn't a weight loss book, and I was never really focused on weight loss to begin with. I am small framed, and weight has never been an ongoing issue for me. Food anxiety and an unhealthy body image, however, have definitely plagued me, and that was something I was trying to tackle head-on. I wanted joy and confidence surrounding my experience with food, and that is why mindfulness became one of the four pillars for the weekly plan.

My favorite part of regular souping is how it makes me feel. It's a lot like my mom's philosophy of letting go. There are some not-so-great elements (sure, call them impurities) in my physical world, and many of them are in my food. I take a full day to let go of unnatural packaged food and overseasoned restaurant food. I pile more fresh vegetables into my diet with daily Soup Swaps where I replace a breakfast, lunch, or dinner with soup. I embrace a simpler food that makes digestion easier for my body and keeps me satisfied longer. And every soup is an opportunity to dive into a ritual that reconnects my emotions and intentions with my physical body and actions. This ritual illuminates me as an active participant in my well-being. It grants me a pause and shows me the work I am doing to take care of myself. It helps me take pride in my actions as they happen and see clearly that I am a strong, confident person.

The act of really focusing on the meal in front of you may seem like an add-on, but this mindful ritual is an integral part of success. Actions only matter as much as we are committed to them, and mindfulness rituals truly establish that commitment. And it doesn't have to be complicated. It's as

(continued on page 16)

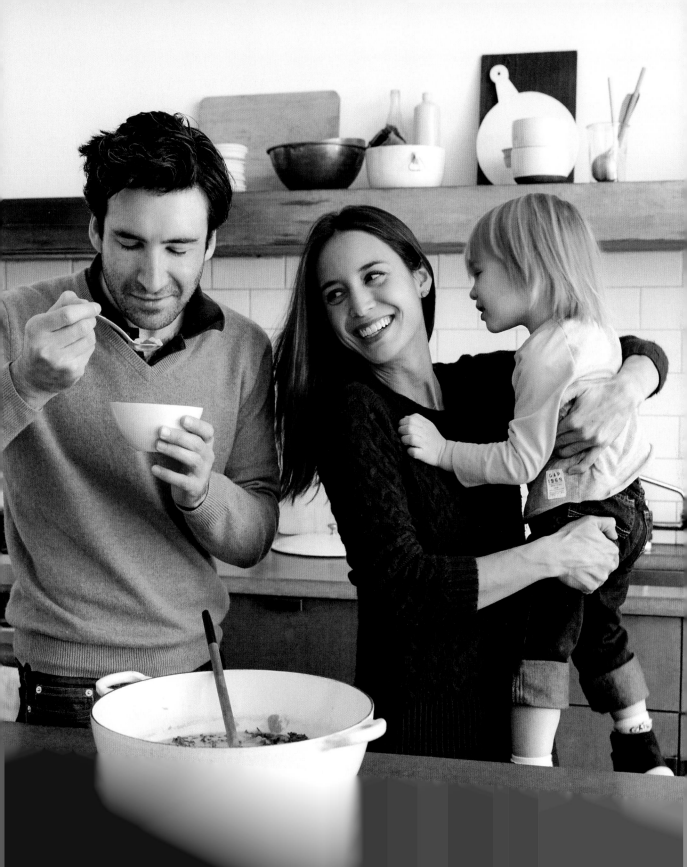

the four pillars of souping

1. **PLANT-BASED NUTRITION.** The Standard American Diet is a little sad: oversaturated in calories and highly refined foods and low in nutrient-dense fruits, vegetables, grains, and legumes. Plants are rich in antioxidants that trap cancer-causing free radicals. They reduce inflammation and fight against diabetes. Plants also reduce oxidative stress (what happens when your body can't keep up with those toxic free radicals pestering your cells) and can even improve your mood. That's why every physician encourages patients to incorporate more vegetables into their diets. But it isn't always easy. Soups are a fantastic solution because cooking concentrates large volumes of vegetables into smaller, easy-to-digest portions while keeping you fuller longer and providing a balance of the vitamins and nutrients you need. Slow-cooking vegetables increases the bioavailability (the amount that your body can use) of fat-soluble vitamins and nutrients like beta-carotene; lycopene; and vitamins K, D, and E. And healthy fats, like olive oil, help your body absorb these nutrients and more readily reap their benefits.

2. **PRACTICALITY.** Convenience and flexibility matter a lot when it comes to sticking to any healthy eating plan. No one wants to be cooking for days, and we all like the freedom to indulge sometimes. A lot of diet programs out there require you to clean out your entire kitchen and overhaul your existing routines. Ready-to-eat food boxes and meal plans can be expensive and are often inflexible because

they rely on foods that must be eaten within a short window of time. Historically, there has been an all-or-nothing mentality when it comes to healthy eating. It really doesn't have to be so extreme. You can choose to make small changes that you can stick to and that make your life easier. It helps to be realistic about just how much change you can make, and the nice thing is, you don't have to make enormous changes to impact your health in a really positive way. I know what it's like when the baby is crying, the e-mail inbox is overflowing, and you can't remember the last time you had a moment for yourself (or a shower, for that matter). The Soup Cleanse is about adopting small changes that make a big difference and are practical for a busy life.

3. **INTERMITTENT FASTING.** Intermittent fasting has been proven to boost metabolism, refresh immunity, detoxify the organs, and shed unwanted weight. By lowering your caloric intake gradually throughout the week, you allow your body to rest and renew. This point can sound a little scary because it feels restrictive to talk about calories. I like to tell it like it is, though, because I know how smart my customers and readers are: We know that calories do count when it comes to maintaining a healthy weight. The point is to become more in touch with the right balance of energy for your body and your lifestyle. I absolutely believe that you should be able to enjoy things like (gasp) refined sugar and baked treats and french fries on occasion. I don't believe in mak-

ing lists of foods that are permanently off-limits. I do think there are a lot of environmental temptations to eat treats more frequently than is good for my health. I rely on my souping routine to keep the indulgences just that and not part of my regular habits. By sticking to a weekly routine with 1 day of souping and 5 days of one soup meal swap, I include intermittent fasting into my week without feeling deprived. The Soup Cleanse Plan incorporates enough lean, plant-based eating to make a difference in anyone's health.

4. **MINDFULNESS.** It feels nice to appreciate the nourishment your body receives! Souping isn't a crash diet. It's embracing a new way of life, a little something I like to call your Splendid Self. It's all about living fully as a participant in your own life. After all, your existence is not a spectator sport. It's about relishing each meal as it nourishes you from the inside out and taking time to savor every sip or spoonful. It's about slowing down and creating small moments of calm in the midst of a hurried life, with less screen time, more playtime, and lots of spooning. Restoring balance in your life doesn't mean juggling a matcha latte and green juice. You need a simple plan with easy-to-use tools that will help you find true Zen. I worked with several meditation experts to create mindful moments for you to use as you soup. These moments are included throughout the recipe pages and will increase your focus and mental strength. Regular mindfulness practice has been proven to make your brain stronger and bigger. It reduces psychological stress, sharpens memory processes, and improves cognitive function. The benefits of mindfulness

aren't just in the brain. It's been shown to strengthen your immune system and even benefit your cardiovascular health!

Bonus: Plant-based meals help us tread a little more lightly on the earth. We stay connected to who we are and to the ground beneath our feet by acknowledging how our food choices affect the world around us. By eating more plants and less meat, we can help reduce environmental pollution caused by animal agriculture. Since having kids, I have become even more passionate about doing my part to leave a healthier planet for future generations. Animal agriculture uses a lot of water—one of earth's precious resources that is in short supply. A whopping 1,800 gallons of water (the equivalent of taking 120 showers) go into a single pound of beef. Compare that to 14 gallons for a pound of carrots, 20 for a pound of spinach, and 40 for a pound of cauliflower, kale, or Brussels sprouts.[14] Much of the meat and dairy Americans eat comes from industrialized agriculture and factory farming, where the use of harmful pesticides, fertilizers, and antibiotics is commonplace. Contamination of the soil, air, and groundwater is an unfortunate by-product of making highly processed animal-based foods. It's nasty stuff, and I really don't like to dwell on it. Instead, I choose to focus on embracing habits that help me become less dependent on animal protein because even little changes make a big difference on my environmental impact.

Every day you eat totally plant-based foods, you reduce your share of greenhouse gas emissions by 75 percent.[15] Every time I soup, I make a difference by saving water and shrinking my carbon footprint (without skipping any showers).

simple as creating a ritual and repeating it. You already do this more or less with your meals by eating them at the same dinner table each evening, at the same time. Here's an opportunity to make that experience richer and more beneficial to building a better you.

The beauty of regular mindfulness is that it opens up new neural connections, strengthening the ones that help us move toward feelings of satisfaction, pride, and happiness. Mindfulness practice makes a real difference on your body,[16] and as your reward centers are stimulated, you will be more and more likely to repeat these exercises. Over time, you may notice that your pace has become more even, that you are more likely to choose to sit down and eat slowly instead of rushing to a meeting. One afternoon while sitting in traffic you may see your emotional state move seamlessly from irritation with the honking truck in front of you to placid appreciation of a song on the radio. You may find your head is less busy with questions and what-ifs and more focused on the present moment.

Starting a new mindfulness ritual may sound daunting, but when you combine it with eating (something that we have to do several times a day anyway), it feels doable. When there's a promise

that it will benefit the whole body, then it starts to feel enticing. And when there's a promise that it will ultimately make your entire life more peaceful, balanced, and enjoyable—does that sound too good to be true? It's real. Mindfulness helped me launch my business, have two completely drug-free births, and find genuine enjoyment in balancing early motherhood and my career as a start-up CEO. When I started connecting mindfulness to my Soup Cleanse Plan, it became so incorporated into my weekly life that it created an inner peace. Connecting mindfulness to food is a bit of a shortcut because you are connecting it to an action that must happen every day, so you are setting yourself up for a much greater chance of success than if you tried to start a mindfulness practice as a stand-alone habit. I will never let go of my mindfulness practice.

I include very simple mindful moments and mantras throughout this book. I also include mindful movements that you can add to your weekly mantras as you branch out and strengthen your souping practice and deepen your connection to yourself. The key to success is uniting yourself with these rituals so they aren't a task you have to check off a list; they just become a part of the natural rhythm of your day.

Souping for Health:
The Weekly Soup Cleanse Plan

This book is shaped around a 7-day plan, but you can tailor it to suit your needs. If you enjoy higher-intensity workouts, I'll show you soup recipes for strength and energy. If you can't stand beans or if you want to limit your salt intake or if you are an expecting mom, I'll show you the best way to soup. My souping plans are rooted in science that shows that regular periods of lean, plant-based eating

keep our bodies healthier and stronger and that in societies eating this way today, people live longer and are more often disease-free. By reconnecting with a more natural rhythm of eating, you'll be tapping into your body's innate power to heal itself and stay your fittest. It means you'll feel awesome, your pants will always button, and you won't be preoccupied with "good" and "bad" foods or dos and don'ts. Souping simplifies your life so you can go on being your Splendid Self.

All of the soup recipes in this book take less than 30 minutes of active cooking time, and every single one of them can be made ahead, stored for later, and used in the weekly Soup Cleanse Plan. The plan lets you mix and match to your heart's content, or you can pick recipes and Soup Cleanse regimens that are targeted for specific health needs. You can switch it up seasonally, taking inspiration from our seasonal calendar, or you can stick to your favorites year-round and swap in something new every so often. The Soup Cleanse program is built around the life of a modern woman. It simplifies your life and strengthens your health so you have a sound foundation to support your best self.

The following 7-day plan is my tried-and-true rhythm, and it's what works for thousands of Splendid Spoon customers, too. It is anchored by a cleanse day and sustained by subsequent days of what I call Soup Swaps. The overall effect is a decrease in weekly calories, an increase in nutrient-dense plant-based food, and high satisfaction. When you combine it with intentional mindful moments, you become even stronger and more con-nected to your rituals, revealing a beautiful sense of confidence and pride in yourself.

- DAY 1: Cleanse. Five soups throughout the day to create a hard reset for mind and body. Soup, soup, and only soup.

- DAYS 2 TO 6: Swap a hearty bowl of soup for one meal per day. Any soup from my recipe col-lection, any meal (though we're partial to lunch, but more on that later). I'll give you tips to make the most of each swap.

- DAY 7: Take a break! Pause, appreciate, have a glass of wine. Kick back, baby. Ever heard the

phrase, If you love something, let it go? It's trite but true. Believe it or not, this is the day that will keep you on track.

You can go for a harder reset with a 2- or 3-day cleanse once every 3 months throughout the year (see the Weight Loss Soup Cleanse Plan in Chapter 3 on page 42), but the 7-day plan will be what works for most of you. These days I don't worry about leaping into a dish of spinach and artichoke dip. I don't worry because I allow myself indul-gences every so often, and I stick to a rhythm each and every week. For most of us, it can be a bit of a kick in the pants to do a 1-day cleanse for the first time, and the daily Soup Swaps will keep you in line thereafter. After the day of rest, you get right back into it. The rhythm is reliable and simple, and it works. It lets you be you, and it keeps you feeling right. For me that means:

- Soup Cleanse Day is a 100 percent me day! "I'm souping" means don't offer me a croissant; keep me off the margarita invite list; and, no, I do not care for a sweet treat at 4 p.m. I actually use the cleanse day as my lazy day. I don't have to think about my food at all because it's premade and lined up, ready to go every 2 hours. I don't go to the gym on this day. I take a bath and drink tea on this day. I go to bed early on this day—and I sleep like a rock.

- I share breakfast and dinner with my kids at least 5 days a week. I don't feel guilty about taco night or make-your-own-pizza night or after-dinner drinks with my girlfriends.

- I feel energized every day. I am confident in myself because every week is rooted in sound plant-based choices. No, I don't eat plant-based all the time, but I know at least 1 full day and five meals after that are super clean and close to ideal.

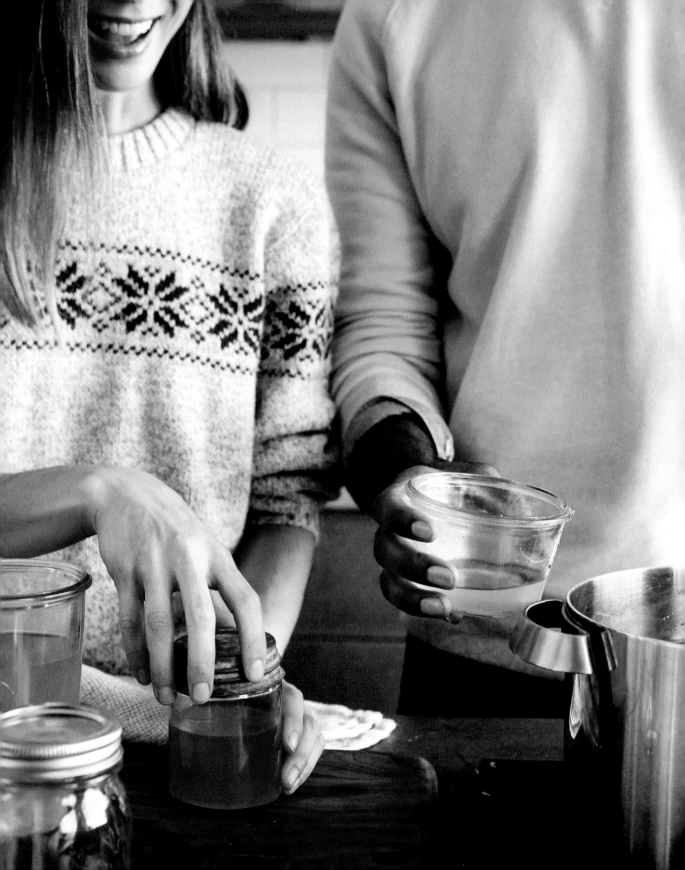

I have to emphasize the best part of this whole plan. After a month of following it, I stopped craving processed foods and I chose meat less (or not at all) when eating out. I also cooked mostly plant-based when I made meals for my kids. In the process of simplifying my diet, my body seemed to be shifting more readily into an even and more natural pace. There were no more manic cravings, and I no longer asked myself permission to have an almond croissant. These days, I rarely choose the almond croissant, so if I want one, I know it's fine and don't feel a crumb of guilt when I'm done.

Regardless of the soups you choose for your soup plan, you should be aware of your daily nutritional needs and goals. And before making any changes to your diet, consult with your doctor, especially if you are trying to lose a significant amount of weight. The Soup Cleanse program works by decreasing your caloric intake through a single day of souping and then meal replacements throughout the week. You're eating real, cooked food made from whole vegetables, so you're giving yourself some of the purest, most readily digestible nutrients you can.

If you are trying to lose weight, there are several quick and easy techniques you can implement to enhance your plan. If you are concerned about your salt intake, I'll show you how you can optimize flavor without adding too much salt. I'll also give a brief overview of the different health benefits of each cleanse regimen: Energize, Heal, Strengthen, Detox, and Weight Loss. And since I'm a mom and I count on a toddler scrambling onto my lap to share everything I bring to the table, I'll show you which recipes are best for moms-to-be and your little ones (those for Mom and Baby).

There are loads of external factors in our world today that have distracted us from a very natural way of eating. Amazingly, it takes just 4 weeks to get back into the true rhythms that will help you achieve your ideal body weight, improve your immune system, increase your energy, and lower your likelihood for heart disease, diabetes, cancer, and a whole host of other ailments. And you don't have to change your life to reap the benefits. You're already doing it. This book will just help you do it better. Harness your Splendid Self and don't look back.

Why Soup?

You soup, she soups, we all soup together. Minestrone, congee, consommé, borscht, sabao, stew, chili—every corner of the earth, every palate, every diet has a soup in it. Soup was probably the first thing our hunter-gatherer ancestors made after they discovered fire, and since then, stirring together a pot of warm victuals has been as natural and soothing as sitting in front of a roaring fire. Soup is a panacea, it's a memory, it's comfort, it's life-giving.

Soup is also remarkably formulated to keep you fuller longer. It's no surprise that your slender and chic great aunt has soup as a first course for every dinner. You eat less if you have soup before a larger meal. There's the famous roast chicken study. A roast chicken with vegetable sides and a glass of water is set before a group of people. The same dinner and water is blended and set before a second group of people as a bowl of soup. Guess which dinner party reported feeling full first and consumed fewer calories? Soup has a profound effect on what is called gastric emptying.[17] Suffice it to say, you feel fuller, longer with soup. Perhaps this is why soup is prevalent in every society and has been since the beginning of time: It's economical. It's no coincidence that soup is the first food made in a time of famine.

Soup is also incredibly flexible because it is an

entire category of food. As you'll see from the variety in this book, soup can be made from just about any vegetable. It can be light and spicy like the Jalapeño Tomato Broth (page 187), and it can be rich and creamy like the Spring Pea with Cashew Cream (page 82). This flexibility means you can have the satisfaction, the comfort, and the healing properties while still keeping your palate excited. It means that the changing seasons will bring new vegetables to transform your cooking experience and stimulate your curiosity. It means you won't get stuck in a soup rut, because there's always a new puree or stew to try as you assemble your Soup Cleanse Plan.

What to Expect

Anticipate being more connected with yourself. Expect to be more aware of what you are eating and how hungry and full you are. Especially on that first Soup Cleanse Day when you are eating exclusively soup, you'll notice the physical and emotional signs of hunger more than you would on the "no rules" day. Embrace this, and you'll start to distinguish between a true physical hunger cue (growling stomach) and an emotional one (I want to share snacks with my coworkers because we always meet at the vending machine around 2 p.m.). This distinction will be incredibly powerful, and it will become stronger every week you soup cleanse. As you connect more to your body's natural cues for hunger and fullness, you won't just be aware of your body, you will strengthen it. Your body and mind will become more connected so that on the Wander Day, the connection will kick in to say, Hey, I remember this feeling: I'm full! Or, Hmmm, I'm not actually hungry right now, but I want to eat—could this be an emotional desire to eat? Maybe I'll wait until I feel those physical cues again. Every time you pause to take notice of these cues and make the distinction between physical and emotional, you are strengthening your foundation, establishing true healthy habits.

Expect to have a little more gas, especially if you aren't accustomed to eating plant-based. Every person is different, but it always takes some time to adjust to more vegetables. The complex carbohydrates and fiber found in vegetables and legumes are not digested by the body so they produce gas. But

i'm starving!

True starvation occurs after your body uses up all the fuel in your stomach, then all the glycogen stores in your liver, and all your fat stores. Temporary hunger is not synonymous with starvation. It's a signal from your body to your mind, and it can be triggered by an empty stomach, the sight of a piece of cake, boredom, or a stressful e-mail. Sometimes that feeling means it really is time to eat, and other times it means we need to relax in another way. Hunger is not the enemy. It's a physical cue about your current state, and how you respond to it will determine how much progress you will make with your relationship with food and with yourself. The stress that manifests in association with hunger is our desire to ignore those cues. Try finding a mindful moment or mantra that helps you connect with your inner strength at such times. One of my favorites is on page 185, "Fears are paper tigers."

here's the thing: Your farts get a bad rap. Lots of different carbohydrates and fibers from vegetables increase the diversity of the healthy (good) bacteria in your gut, or microbiota. This diversity keeps our digestive systems sound and has been shown to keep us at a healthier weight. Purna C. Kashyap, a gastroenterologist at the Mayo Clinic, says, "Eating foods that cause gas is the only way for the microbes in the gut to get nutrients. If we didn't feed them carbohydrates, it would be harder for them to live in our gut . . . undigested carbohydrates let the whole [microbiotic] ecosystem thrive and flourish."[18]

On a related note, expect to have more regular bowel movements. Many experience multiple bowel movements on their Soup Cleanse Day. As I'll discuss in Chapter 2, this is due to insoluble fiber. Vegetables have lots of insoluble fiber, and it acts like a broom in your digestive system: This indigestible matter literally cleans you out. If that's not cleansing, I don't know what is. Appreciate your body's ability to let go of all the stuff it simply doesn't need.

Expect to be pleasantly surprised by how satisfied you feel with the routine after 4 weeks or possibly even sooner. You will come to appreciate the soups as comforting and reliable moments throughout your week. You will be able to let go and let the soup do some of the hard work for you in your quest to establish better eating habits. If you stick with the Soup Cleanse program for 4 weeks, I promise that you will feel stronger, more confident, and more grounded.

What If I Cheat?

The whole purpose of the 7-day plan is to eliminate *cheating* from the diet vernacular. There is a lean day (the Soup Cleanse Day), there is a day without rules (Wander), and there are the 5 days in between where you replace a meal a day with soup. You are reducing your caloric intake significantly enough that you should be able to carry on with some (even most!) of your old habits and still see results. After a month, more of the habits that led you astray in the past will fall to the wayside because you will have developed a clear awareness of your actions and a deeper connection to the habits that reward you with good health. You'll start opting for an extra serving of vegetables instead of meatballs at that next family feast.

A month of dedication and you won't be talking about cheating, you'll be focused on feeling your best. You will have your souping day, you will have your soup swaps, you will indulge some, you will get back to your lean day—you will live your life. You will enjoy being an active participant in your good health.

But what if you skip a day? What if you can't cleanse this week? What if you go on vacation? It's okay. The point is just to hop back into it. A skipped day of souping is not the end of the world. A full week of vacation eating isn't ideal, but it's not going to completely derail you. Get back into it and be proud that you are into it. Treat it as an opportunity to reevaluate your recipes, try some new ones, and add variety to your routine. Look at those vacations or prolonged Wander Days as an opportunity to reconnect with why you picked up this book in the first place. Reflection is great for the soul, and it can help us make better decisions as we move forward. We are all about moving forward.

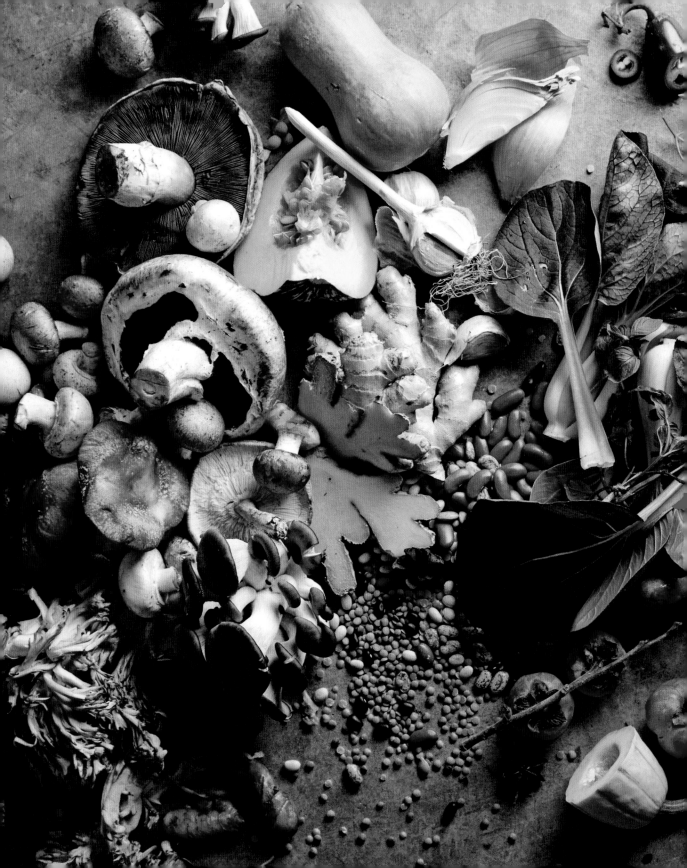

chapter 2

WHY VEGGIES? WHY SOUP?

I'm Not Vegan; I Just Veg a Lot

Living a healthy life isn't about perfection. That's why crash diets fail; why New Year's resolutions go stale by February; and why, despite our fitness- and diet-obsessed culture, our eating habits are sadly lacking diversity and vital nutrients. As I said in the previous chapter, according to the Centers for Disease Control and Prevention, 87 percent of Americans don't meet the daily recommendation for vegetable consumption[1] and nearly 69 percent of adults are overweight or obese.[2] Eating healthy can be intimidating, and the rules seem to change constantly, with the bad-for-you foods shifting like sand. But one constant holds true: We need to eat more fruits and vegetables. They are the best fuel we can give our bodies, they improve our lives from the inside out, and they are why societies who eat primarily plant-based live the longest.[3]

The pressure for us to subscribe 100 percent to a diet or fitness routine is monumental. Gym memberships, health coaches, meal plans, and calorie trackers abound. You can stalk nearly every carb you eat and creep on every calorie you burn, all with the touch of a screen! I try to integrate healthy food choices into my lifestyle, not change my entire lifestyle to accommodate a particular trend or craze. This simply helps me stay sane. I love preparing and eating nutritious, plant-based meals, so I never feel like I have to put my life on hold until I lose however many pounds or fit into that one tauntingly snug pair of jeans. Healthy living has as much to do with the thoughts we think as the food we eat. You don't have to immediately swear off mac 'n' cheese and potato chips forever. Instead, take it meal by meal, asking yourself: What will this food do for me? How will it nourish my body and fuel the projects or activities that I want to do?

Embracing the healthiest you and maintaining that vision for yourself doesn't require that you subscribe to a diet dogma. It's not about being perfect. It's less about what you're removing from your diet and more about what you're adding to it. Think about all of the amazingly delicious, brightly colored, and nutrient-rich foods that you get to eat and how phenomenal they make you feel. Once you fill your plate (or bowl) up with these beauties, you'll realize just how little room you have left for the other stuff. Your appetite and palate will start to shift, and you'll begin craving what your body actually needs.

If your approach to healthy eating is punishment, then you'll always need to "reward" yourself with fatty, salty, and sugary treats that are as nutrient-poor as they are highly processed. Here's a thought: What if you simplified your goals? What if you realized that you could improve the quality of your mind and body with just a few small shifts? Remind yourself that even one plant-based meal a day really does make a difference.

Souper Powers

Souping for health is one of the easiest ways to restart good eating habits, feel great, get fit, or just maintain a healthy weight. I talked about the science of soup previously, so now let's discuss soup's power as a connector to our emotions.

Soup has been around for as long as humans have been cooking.[4] The impulse to throw vegetables into a pot and cook them down into liquid form practically flows through our genetic makeup, and it crosses class and cultural divides.

You can probably remember since childhood helping chop vegetables for a stew or gathering around a steaming pot and watching the delicious ladling of bowls begin. The preparation and consumption of soup encourage sharing and social engagement, an important part of internal and external health. If the bowl is the individual, the kettle is the community. There's something connective about being nourished from the same dish as those you're sharing a meal with.

There's also something about the slowness of soup that creates a unique meditation for me. Most of the recipes in this book require less than 30 minutes of active cooking time, but what about that hour or so of simmering? And what about that phenomenon of soup often tasting better the day after you cook it? I like to imagine the ingredients transforming throughout the cooking process. Garlic is a dense bulb containing the potential to grow into another garlic plant. I choose to break it open; unlock a clove from the bulb; release it from its paper shell; dice it into countless sticky and pungent pieces, its anticancer enzyme, alliinase, activating in the process. Then, with some heat and a little plant-based fat, those pieces transform from raw and spicy to sweet and delicate. Layer upon layer of flavor and texture are added to the pot,

and then I must step back and let time take over. This is often a welcome relief because I have kids who want to be read to, diapers that need changing, or e-mails asking for answers. Better yet, I have a few yoga poses I want to stretch into, an article I may have otherwise not found time to read, or a friend I'd like to invite to my dinner table.

It's also a reminder to let go. Sometimes, the best thing you can do with soup (and with unanswerable work questions, a trying situation with a toddler, or a lost set of keys) is step back and let go. Let the soup simmer on its own, let your toddler figure out his zipper, let those keys stay lost for a few more minutes. In life, and with soup, you do the best you can with the recipe and ingredients you have, and at a certain point, you have to let gravity take over. The world keeps spinning, and when it's time to take the soup off the burner, you'll know. And your patience will be rewarded.

Soup has lots of tangible benefits that I'll continue to talk about below. Soup's ability to help me slow down, to reconnect me with the transformative process of cooking, and to shift my perspective from "when will this be done" to "I have an open moment in my day" is perhaps its most mysterious and enchanting power.

Let's Heat Things Up

Let's bring it back down to earth for a moment so I can tell you about some of those nutrition elements that make soup so special. The moment food is harvested from the ground it begins to lose nutrients. That's why purchasing fresh, local fruits and vegetables is better for you. It's one of the reasons I make it a priority at Splendid Spoon. But cooking doesn't necessarily speed up that process. In many instances, it's quite the opposite. Did you know

that slow-cooking certain vegetables releases more nutrients than if you ate them raw? The notion that raw is better than cooked because heating food will kill vital nutrients isn't totally true. While some plants experience a decrease in certain vitamins when heated, others nearly explode with increased nutrients and antioxidants because of it. Vitamin C is one that gets quickly zapped when cooked, but it can easily be found elsewhere in abundance, like in citrus fruits, kiwifruit, and leafy salad greens, all delicious when eaten raw. It's harder to find the nutrients that emerge from cooked food in a raw form. Lycopene, for example, is available in raw red grapefruit and raw tomatoes, but it is more potent in cooked tomatoes.

The gentle heat of steaming or slow-cooking can release or preserve nutrients in veggies. Plus, consuming cooked vegetables along with good fat, such as olive oil, aids in the absorption of fat-soluble vitamins like A, E, D, and K.[5] Much depends on the solubility of the vitamins and nutrients. Vitamins are either water-soluble or fat-soluble. Water-soluble vitamins, such as vitamin C, are easily lost when cooked, as they are more fragile. They can be easily eradicated through heat or leeched into the cooking water. Fat-soluble vitamins are in it for the long haul. They are dissolved in fat and then stored in your body tissue, which means they are more durable and can take a hit from the burner's flame.

Let's think of cooking (especially slow-cooking) as an external part of the digestive process. It's already doing the work of breaking down your food, saving your jaw a lot of strain, and making it easier for you to chew and ingest. Foods like grains and legumes are basically impossible to eat raw (and at the very least, not as enjoyable). Not only does cooking food make it physically easier for you to eat, but it also makes many ingredients better for you by allowing their nutrients to be more easily absorbed. Here are some nutrients that remain stable when cooked and how they benefit your body.

Lycopene

Do you know what gives tomatoes (and other crimson-hued veggies) their beautifully rich red color? It's called lycopene, a phytochemical (this just means a compound made naturally by plants). Lycopene boasts antioxidant superpowers and is a ninja at trapping cancer-causing free radicals in our food. Free radicals are anything but radical. They naturally occur during digestion, but they can foster dangerous cancer cells if they aren't combated by foods that are rich in antioxidants. Did you know that cooking tomatoes just 30 minutes increases trans-lycopene content by 164 percent and raises antioxidant levels by 62 percent compared with raw consumption?[6]

SOUP SPOTLIGHT: Cooked gazpacho? You bet. Instead of sticking to the traditional raw preparation, I like to light a fire under my tomatoes for this summery soup (see page 62). Then I let it chill out, and enjoy as usual.

Vitamin A

We all know carrots are great for our eyes, but did you know their vitamin A superstar beta-carotene could also reduce the risk of cancer and depression?[7] Just one carrot contains 210 percent of your daily dose of vitamin A in the form of beta-carotene. Talk about eye candy! Munching down on carrots Bugs Bunny–style is fine and dandy, but if you want to increase your antioxidant levels and fight the good fight against ocular cell damage, put these beauties in a pot.[8] When cooked, the level of carotenoids increases, thus allowing you to absorb more antioxidants with each bite.[9] Keep calm and carrot on.

SOUP SPOTLIGHT: Carrot and Turmeric soup on page 81 is a great way to start the day and awaken your eyes with something made just for them. This recipe is rich in antioxidants and vitamin A, along with turmeric to get your circulation pumping. Fresh carrots set your eyes a-shinin'. Citrus gets your taste buds dancin'. A dash of ground red pepper adds a lively kick to get you out the door and on your way.

Vitamin D

Vitamin D is critical for our health because it works hand in hand with calcium to help our bodies integrate that calcium into our bones. Vitamin D is also linked to our moods, with more and more studies revealing that individuals experiencing depression are deficient in this nutrient. Sunshine is where most of us get our dose, but supposedly 1 billion people globally are lacking enough of this feel-good vitamin.[10] (More reason for dining al fresco!) Fungi are the only nonanimal source to provide vitamin D naturally, and since heat doesn't reduce any of its power, I love to include mushrooms in my soups.

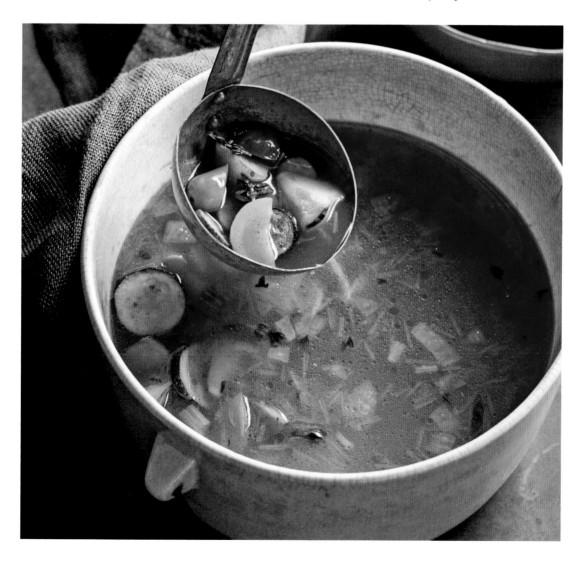

SOUP SPOTLIGHT: Bringing the flavors of the classic dish chicken with rice to life in a fully plant-based form was my inspiration behind "Chicken" Stew with Rice on page 161. I slice up big oyster mushrooms because their flesh is the perfect texture to (nearly) fool even the meatiest of meat-lovers. There's something about sinking your teeth into those mushrooms and slurping that hot broth that makes you sit back and appreciate the power of soup. Maybe because it reminds me of the chicken soup my mom used to make me, or maybe it's those endorphins kicking in from all that 'shroomy vitamin D. If that's a placebo effect, I don't mind, because I know that vitamin D is hitting my bloodstream soon enough.

Vitamin K

Like vitamin D, vitamin K remains stable when heated, and it is fat soluble, meaning your body needs a fat to transport it to the cells that need it most. It is also essential to blood health. And when you think about blood as the medium that transports nutrients and oxygen to where they need to go (while also moving toxins, like carbon dioxide, toward their exit routes), it's a wonder we don't talk more about the health of our blood. Specifically, vitamin K makes sure our blood clots when it needs to, and it assists in calcium transport through the bloodstream. The healthy bacteria in our gut naturally make vitamin K, and greens in the cruciferous family—like broccoli, kale, and collards—supply it. Those cruciferous greens are also a great source of the

dietary fiber that the healthy gut bacteria flourish on. Don't you love when things come full circle like that?

SOUP SPOTLIGHT: Who says leafy greens have to be tough? Curly Kale Stew on page 149 features sweet and tart tomatoes, creamy coconut milk, and the rich and complex flavor of Madras curry. You'll be licking your bowl.

Vitamin E

Vitamin E is an essential vitamin for clear and bright skin and is often included in topical creams. It's a powerful antioxidant that strengthens you from the inside, as well, and it is not affected by heat. Since vitamin E is fat soluble, we make sure to combine vitamin E–containing plants with healthy fats, like olive oil, avocado, and coconut oil. Actually, some of the richest sources of vitamin E have higher concentrations of plant-based fats in them already, such as sunflower seeds, walnuts, and almonds. Vitamin E has excellent anti-inflammatory properties, which means it is a big boon to your immune system, will help you recover from injury, and generally keeps your cells in great shape.

SOUP SPOTLIGHT: There's no shortage of rich flavor in Plant-Based Tagine on page 103. This North African–inspired dish features chickpeas, cocoa powder, and apricots. The almonds in this recipe are high in vitamin E—and crunch, something you don't always expect in a soup. The digestive fluids in your mouth benefit from that crunching motion, too.

Fiber: The Original Superfood

Fiber is one of nature's simplest and most powerful friends to the human body. It is essentially a matrix of indigestible parts of the plant, but when set in

motion by the digestive system, it helps the whole body run smoother, faster, and stronger. The American diet is sadly deficient in fiber. We consume a

slow down and chew your food

Chew, chew, chew. It's what we're told growing up, but it's not always easy to integrate mindful chewing into our mealtime habits (check out page 169 for a mindful chewing exercise with the crunchy chia seeds found in the Avocado Kimchi Stew). Fibrous foods are great in that they basically demand to be chewed thoroughly, allowing us time to gauge our level of fullness as it occurs, not afterward, when the food coma has already set in. Slowing down consumption and increasing awareness of satiety contribute to weight loss and establishing mindful eating habits.

daily average of only 15 of the 20 to 35 grams needed,[11] and our hunter-gatherer ancestors ate an estimated 10 times the amount of fiber we do today (and we thought we were so evolved!).

All fiber is made up of carbohydrates, but our bodies cannot break them down, so we don't absorb those calories. Eating a high-fiber diet can help you shed unwanted weight because you feel fuller for longer while accelerating the digestive process. Fiber comes in two forms: soluble and insoluble.

Soluble fiber works to slow down digestion, allowing the body time to break down and absorb the nutrients in foods. This fiber dissolves in water, transforming into a gel-like substance in your stomach, giving you a feeling of fullness. Soluble fiber is what gives you staying power when you eat a bowl of oatmeal or a lentil stew and, in turn, helps keep your meal portions in check. For folks with diabetes, the gel-like substance that soluble fiber creates in the stomach slows down the release of sugar into the bloodstream, keeping glucose levels from spiking. Plus, soluble fiber clears our vascular networks of unhealthy plaques, keeping our blood pressure low and improving overall circulation and oxygenation to our organs.[12]

Insoluble fiber is like the hyperactive twin, speeding up digestion and pushing your meal along its journey through your digestive and intestinal tracts. Insoluble fiber comes from the rigid cellulose in plant cells, and it gives the plant structure.

While it goes without saying that insoluble fiber keeps things running smoothly and eliminates constipation, digestion isn't this fiber's only line of work. Insoluble fiber plays a significant role in maintaining balance in the microbiota, or flora, of our guts. All the "good" bacteria that live in our bellies feast on that insoluble fibrous matter. Healthy gut microbiota can prevent everything from allergies and skin afflictions to cancers and weight gain.

When dietary fiber is increased, microbial profiles related to obesity shift to those found in leaner physiques. We can't digest fibrous matter, but our gut bacteria sure love it. Good microbes thrive on fermentable fiber, and if we don't feed them properly, they quickly turn to devouring the mucus that lines and protects our gut from disease and inflammation. Our friendly gut microbes have the ability to tease out unused energy, vitamins, nutrients, and fatty acids stored in fiber.

Soluble fiber is found in nuts, seeds, legumes, beans, peas, oats, and barley. Insoluble fiber is a part of every plant cell, and so it is found in literally every vegetable and fruit. Many fiber-rich foods contain both kinds of fiber, working together to maintain a natural balance in your body's digestion.

As I mentioned earlier in the "What to Expect" section in Chapter 1, souping will probably get your system, ahem, moving more frequently than you are accustomed to. This is a good thing, but I totally get that it can be a little weird, embarrassing, or even uncomfortable. All the Soup Cleanse programs have both soluble and insoluble fiber in them. The recipes for Weight Loss will have more fiber than others, and the recipes for Mom and Baby will have a little less. I also include a healthy dose of fat in my recipes, not only for taste and satiety but also because digesting high-fiber foods with fat will reduce bloating and cramping.

Plant Power

Not every vegetable is created equally. Some are packed with heart-friendly, cholesterol-lowering, and tummy-shrinking nutrients. And then some are essentially green water with some crunch around the edges. Knowing the mighty from the "meh" is important when grocery shopping for plant power. Here are some of my favorite veggies, herbs, and spices to help you get started. Don't waste your time or money on chopping up iceberg lettuce and celery sticks when you can enjoy a hearty, colorful, and vibrant selection of ingredients that will taste as good as they are for you.

LEAFY GREENS. Kale, Swiss chard, bok choy, spinach—these leafy greens are all rich sources of vitamin K, vitamin A, and the sulfur-containing compounds that help diversify the healthy bacteria colonies in your gut.

BRIGHTLY HUED VEGETABLES. Tomatoes, peppers, summer squash, eggplant—these vegetables come in a variety of shades, and every color has a slightly different phytonutrient profile. Try orange bell peppers, speckled eggplant, and yellow tomatoes, and enjoy the unique benefits of each.

LEGUMES. Black beans, pinto beans, fava beans, and lentils are all part of the legume family. They are one of the best sources of protein for a plant-based diet. Their mix of protein and soluble fiber is what helps them have great staying power, and it's why legume-based soups are featured earlier in the day for the Soup Cleanse Day.

ROOT VEGETABLES. Root vegetables like yams, celeriac, and carrots are literally the root system of the plant—pulling nutrients out of the soil and delivering them into the body of the plant. For this reason, there are high concentrations of nutrients just below the skin. Go for younger root vegetables or those with a thin skin whenever possible and skip the peeler.

FRESH HERBS. Fresh herbs are the secret ingredient to creating depth in every spoonful. Delicate herbs like basil, mint, chive, and parsley are best chopped and sprinkled at the end. This is my favorite way to add a burst of freshness to just about any soup. The hardier, woody-stemmed herbs, like rosemary and thyme, are lovely during the base-building process and will make your kitchen smell like Provence. Oh la la!

MUSHROOMS. Oyster, shiitake, enoki—I've never met a mushroom I didn't like. They release loads of powerful flavor molecules when mixed with a bit of fat and roasted or sautéed, and they create the trademark "meaty" flavor in many of my soups.

Some people just don't love mushrooms; if it's the texture that bothers you, just strain or scoop out the mushrooms before eating so you get their flavor in the broth. If they turn you off completely, you can replace mushrooms with chunks of roasted sweet squash (the sweet and earthy flavor of squash is about as close as you can get to the unique mushroom flavor without using mushrooms). Or simply add more of the other vegetables in the recipe.

SPIRULINA. This is an emerald-colored powder made up of dried sea algae. It's valued for its concentration of nutrients like protein, iron, and calcium. Because it is high in nutrition and low in volume, spirulina is an easy add-in to boost the profile of the broths without adding a lot more fibrous vegetables. Plus, your soup will take on a beautiful deep-green hue. If you can't find it in a health food store, you can always just add some extra spinach or use dried seaweed.

GROUND GREEN TEA (MATCHA). I love matcha, similar to spirulina, for its concentration of antioxidants. It's one of my favorite additions to soups containing fruit because it tempers a fruit's sweet flavor with a little bitterness to create a more sophisticated profile. It has caffeine, too, so be aware that you might get an extra jolt of productivity out of matcha-containing soups.

HEMPSEED. This seed is considered a perfect protein because of its amino acid profile and the ratio of omega-3 to omega-6 (heart-healthy) fats. I love it because it's yet another seed that has become more readily available at the grocery store, and it's fun to try new ingredients. Hempseed has a very light texture and just a whisper of the trademark pungent, skunky flavor that you think of with cannabis.

SAIGON CINNAMON. Not all cinnamon is created equal. Saigon cinnamon, also known as Vietnamese cinnamon, comes from the bark of a different plant variety (cassia) than conventional or Ceylon cinnamon, which is a "true" cinnamon plant. In studies, Saigon cinnamon has been shown to have positive effects on cardiovascular health, whereas Ceylon cinnamon has not. I use it for flavor, too, so if you can't find Saigon (which has a slightly more intense flavor), use what you have in your cabinet and feel free to be a little more liberal with seasoning.

TURMERIC. The rhizome, part of a plant's root structure, is what you are eating when you add turmeric to your soups. This bright orange superfood is loaded with anti-inflammatory compounds. The best way to access those compounds is by adding heat and a little black pepper. I love fresh turmeric, but you can use dry, as well. Expect the fresh stuff to color your fingertips and countertops; the pigment in turmeric practically glows orange and is what gives curry its color.

READY? LET'S GO! I counted the calories so you don't have to. The 7-day Soup Cleanse Plan is designed to reduce calories and increase satiety, helping you feel your best and reach your wellness and weight loss goals. At its core are 10 soups that you enjoy over the week. Those soups replace a number of your higher-calorie meals while estab-lishing an easy-to-follow rhythm and building a stronger foundation for your healthiest self. The results are an increase in nutrition, stronger healthy habits, and a simplified routine.

The road map for the 7-day Soup Cleanse Plan looks like this.

1 Day a Week: **Cleanse**

Soup all day. You'll have five soups throughout this leaner-than-most day to detox your body and boost digestion. This is a day all about you. It's a great day to slow down, so I suggest using it as a rest day from your typical exercise routine, as well. You'll be getting a mix of physical and mental or emotional cues as you soup all day. Let this help you be present and mindful of your experience.

Part 2 of this book is designed to provide you with recipes in the order that you will eat them on this lean day: Your heartiest, most protein- and fat-dense soups will be earlier in the day; followed by a mix of hearty and light soups of various tex-tures; and you'll finish with a warm broth to put your body at ease before you rest. The cleanse day shouldn't be incredibly difficult, but it's an adjust-ment for most, and that's normal. It's a rhythm our ancestors were accustomed to, but we've also had many years of super-convenient, nutrient-deficient, calorie-dense food at our fingertips. The lean soup day is much easier than any other cleanse or fast I've done in the past, but it's not always easy. This is a day that will push your body a bit, and in return you will become stronger.

Here are some tips to get back in touch with your ancestral biology.

1. WAKE UP WITH 10 DEEP BREATHS AND TOE-TO-SKY STRETCHES. This is a great start to your day and a wonderful way to stretch and move between soups. Do it as often as you want. The oxygen from deep breathing energizes your brain, relaxes your muscles, and evens out your heart rate. You don't have to be a seasoned yogi to take advantage of the head-clearing benefits of deep breathing and stretching. Breathe in fully, allowing your lungs to fill completely with air, and raise your arms to the sky. Wiggle your fingers to greet the sun even if you can't see it. Then bring your arms down and bend from your waist as you exhale and touch your shins or your toes or the ground; you want to feel a stretch, not a strain. Let your body hang natu-rally like a limp rag doll and feel the sleep shake out of your muscles. Raise your body up again and greet the day. Repeat until you've stretched through 10 big breaths.

2. UNWIND WITH A HEAD-TO-TOE BODY SCAN. Feeling stressed or anxious? Just realize you forgot to mail your credit card bill last month? Feeling like you have to have something other than soup before you go into that big meeting? Feeling like your body might take over and bring you to the vending machine? Give your-self 5 minutes to connect to your emotional state and the physical manifestations of those emotions in your body. This is a calming exer-

cise that you can do whenever you feel a little off balance. Find a quiet place and close your eyes for 5 minutes. Take three deep breaths, filling your lungs with air, holding your breath for a blink, and then exhaling slowly. Starting from the top of your head, slowly move through your body and acknowledge your physical and emotional state. Move through your forehead and acknowledge how scrunched it is—let it go. Move down to your jaw and acknowledge that it may be clenched or tense—let it go. Scan through your shoulder blades and feel the tingling sensation of your stress as knots—let them go. And so on. This is a really powerful exercise! The first few times you might get distracted, but be easy on yourself and gently bring your focus back to scanning your body. This is a form of meditation that will relax you. Your body will thank you by "remembering" this exercise the next time it's in stress mode. Before you know it, you will be sitting at your desk, feel a knot, and take a moment to let it go. That's when your practice has become a real part of you, and your body has begun to release stress in a truly healthy way.

3. GET OUTSIDE! Embrace your inner cavegirl and get outside for some fresh air. Take a stroll and enjoy the sun or wind on your skin. We aren't meant to be inside all day. Warm up with your soup in a thermos and spoon outdoors, or pour it over ice on a steamy day and sit in the shade while you sip. The physical sensation of the breeze on your face and the crunch of leaves underfoot will help ground you deeper into your souping experience and your relationship with your body and the world around you.

4. PACE YOURSELF. Pay attention to how full you are between soups. If you have half a bowl of soup and feel full, that's great. Wrap up your leftover soup and allow yourself to go back to that half bowl in about an hour. Keep herbal tea on hand and enjoy a warm mug between your soups.

5. DRINK YOUR COFFEE: IT'S A-OK. Coffee has been proven time and again to be a rich source of antioxidants and to help improve focus. Heck, I even put it in a few soup recipes! Have a cup in the morning if that's your typical routine. Or have one after your first soup. Keep it black or add a dash of almond milk, but no dairy, please. Remember, your cavegirl self was foraging on those lean days, with no pet goats or cows to give her milk.

6. SKIP THAT GLASS OF WINE. I know I said this is a day all about you, and you love to unwind from the chaos of the day with a big glass of red. But this is just one day. It's as much about connecting with yourself as it is about abstaining from some of the extras. Alcohol is a source of hidden calories for a lot of us, meaning we often drink it as a beverage and forget that it has a caloric count that influences weight. It also has that boozy effect on our mood and endorphins. Just like we are trying to really understand the cues that have us reaching for food (physical hunger vs. emotional desire), we can take this day to clue ourselves in to why we reach for a glass of wine. This is just one day to say, I'm going to relax in a different way. Unwind with an aromatic bath, let yourself daydream to a new mix, or go get a pedicure. Besides, one glass of red is going to hit your bloodstream like whoa after this lean day of souping!

5 Days a Week: **Swap**

You conquered that cleanse day! Rise and stretch and greet the rest of your week. You woke up feeling refreshed and, surprisingly, not famished. You make breakfast as usual, maybe thinking a little more about what you choose instead of going into autopilot toward a bagel with cream cheese. Or you have that bagel with cream cheese and wonder, Eek, did I just derail myself after all that hard work yesterday?! Don't worry. You are still on track, my friend. When lunch comes, you will have a fresh plant-based soup. You will have a mini cleanse day experience right there at your desk or at home or outside in the sunshine. I recommend swapping out the typical lunch for soup throughout the week because it keeps the habit going. It sweeps in just when you need it: after breakfast and before the dinner you plan to share with your family or have out with friends. It's me time again, even if for only this one meal. That's not to say you should go out of your way to indulge during your other nonsoup meals, but the point is to create a repeatable rhythm that works for *you* and *your* life. The habit is most important.

Think of your soup swap as an anchor in your day to keep you on track. Your hearty bowl of soup brings your vegetable intake up another 3 servings (win!) and keeps your calorie count just a bit lower so you stay on track with your wellness goals without feeling deprived (win! win!). It further strengthens your foundation by building in a reliable habit that's easy to repeat the next 4 days until—wait, is that it?

Here are a few more tips for making the most of your swaps.

1. Choose soups that you really, really love. Yes, it's fine to make a double batch of the Courgette Stew (page 144) and have it every day for lunch!

And no, it doesn't matter if you always pick from one category or another. If you love the purees because you can heat them up and sip them during your working lunches, that's totally fine. One of the great things about soup is that it stores remarkably well in the freezer; the nutrients are preserved just as they were when you made the soup and are ready to nourish you once thawed. Make batches of what you love so you look forward to the plant-based fuel you get with each swap.

2. On that note, it's fine to swap soup for dinner or breakfast if that's your preference. I suggest lunch because this tends to be the easiest meal for most people to stick with throughout the week. Life is easier when you take out the guesswork. If, however, you go out to lunch many days of the week for your job or if that's your quality time with good friends, then the lunch swap may not be best for you. The point is to not make it a "thing." You shouldn't be looking at the calendar every week deciding how to fit your soup swaps into your life. Or if dinner seems to be the meal that consistently throws you off track, maybe it would be a good idea to swap dinner so you can really reconnect with your physical hunger cues again and suss out some of the emotional connections you may have to that meal. The point is, try to pick the meal you can stick to 90 percent of the time, and then line up your soups and go. If you like being flexible on a daily basis, that's fine, too; I just find that sticking to the same meal most of the time is best for habit formation.

3. What about the nonsoup meals? As I've talked about before, a big part of souping is reconnecting with yourself. After 4 weeks, the routine

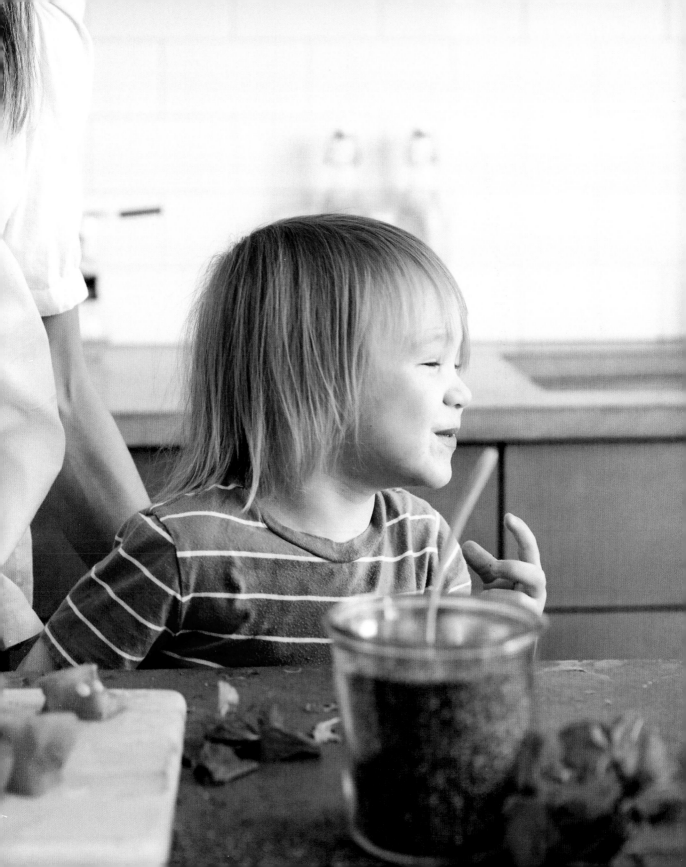

will be a habit and you'll have a much better connection to your unique hunger cues. You will also be better at deciding when you're hungry, when you're not, and which foods will build the best foundation for you. But what about those first 4 weeks? Don't sweat it so much. The point is to create a deeper connection with yourself. The key to long-term healthy eating is to establish real habits that are ingrained in you—and that's not going to happen if you try to change every current habit. Souping is not about immediate perfection. You're making a big shift with a cleanse day and five swaps—congratulate yourself! Have your roast chicken dinner every Thursday night if that's what you do. Don't worry so much about the content of the nonsoup meals those first 4 weeks. Focus, instead, on what your body says to you as you eat. Try to pull your habits from that cleanse day into your swaps and into your other nonsoup meals. And don't be so hard on yourself. You will have another swap tomorrow and another cleanse day in less than a week. Appreciate the present and look forward.

If the Soup Cleanse Day is structural support for the foundation you are building (the soil graded evenly, the holes drilled into the ground, the steel laid in a grid pattern), then the 5 days of swaps are the concrete. The structure has to be there first, or the concrete will form freely all over the place. But with the structure in place, the concrete can flow just right so that it becomes the solid support you want it to be. And once you have that foundation in place, what do you do? You paint it red, baby.

1 Day a Week: **Wander!**

If the cleanse day is the support grid and the swaps are your concrete, then your last day of the week is definitely the paint. It can be what you want because it doesn't change the integrity of the foundation. It's what makes your foundation yours. The Soup Cleanse program includes structure and discipline in the cleanse and meal swaps, but it also acknowledges the beauty of a day without structure. This isn't to say you should go out of your way to consume as much nutrient-deficient processed food as possible. I have a feeling you wouldn't be reading this book if you were that type of gal. The point is, if you are invited to a birthday party and chicken wings and beer are being served, you don't have to bargain with yourself about how much or little you eat for fear it will chip away at the strong foundation you have been building all week.

The simplicity of the Soup Cleanse Plan is that it is flexible—we all don't eat perfectly every day and every meal. The plan is bookended intentionally by a cleanse day and a no-rules day. Taking a break is a good thing! Take pause, appreciate your dedication, and let yourself wander. Take comfort in the fact that your one all-day souping ritual will be there for you tomorrow.

As I mentioned earlier, the core of the plan is 10 total soup meals that are enjoyed throughout the course of your week. Could you do 2 cleanse days back to back and then eat "normally" for the following 5 days? Sure, but I've found that repeating the souping experience throughout the week really keeps people on track and establishes the great habits that will make your foundation strong and help you make even better decisions moving forward.

How to Use This Book

Five recipes from this book give you 20 soup servings, or 2 weeks' worth of soup. As I mentioned earlier, the Soup Cleanse Day is like the iron gridwork that structures your foundation and the swaps are like the concrete that creates the strength of the foundation. Select five recipes based on how you want your Soup Cleanse Day to look; the remaining 15 soup servings will store well in the fridge or freezer so you can easily grab and go for the Soup Swap Days and your second Soup Cleanse Day.

The recipe section is categorized into five chapters. They are organized as follows with the Soup Cleanse Day in mind, because this is the order that will provide the best satisfaction and improve digestion on that day.

1. PUREES: Jump-start your metabolism with a fiber-rich puree.

2. BEANS AND LENTILS: Set yourself up for long-lasting satisfaction with a high-protein/high-fat bean or lentil soup.

3. SWEETER SPOONFULS: Take in a slightly sweeter soup in the afternoon to boost energy without the crash.

4. RESTORATIVE STEWS: Give yourself something hearty to chew for dinner.

5. RESTORATIVE BROTHS: Prime your body for rest with a soothing broth.

Each recipe is labeled to let you know that particular soup has nutrients and micronutrients that can help your body energize, strengthen, detox, lose weight, or heal. I have also labeled which recipes are for mom and baby because I love sharing these soups with my kids. Plus, these have extra nutrients like folic acid and calcium that are great for pregnant and breastfeeding moms, too.

Throughout my time developing recipes and talking with customers, I have found that everyone has preferences, and because soup (and food in general) is so closely tied with memory, many think that the beet puree, for example, will taste like their great aunt's borscht—which they absolutely love (or flat-out despise). I always encourage trying something new or giving your palate a chance to try an ingredient or texture you thought you didn't like. Supposedly you need up to seven attempts to start liking a specific ingredient. So if you haven't had beets since you were in third grade, maybe give them a try again. Who knows, maybe a soup with beets and orange zest will tickle you the right way.

Maybe you haven't had chilled soup before at all—give it a shot! Nearly every other culture in the world has a chilled soup (and I'm not talking just gazpacho)—and think about how many more opportunities you will have to enjoy your soup if you can experience it in two different temperatures. Soup is as cooling in summer as it is warming in winter. What's more, you are that much closer to eating a chilled soup than a warm one because you don't have to reheat it. That said, there's a great amount of variety in this book, so there should be something for everyone, even if you despise beets. And *every* soup can be enjoyed warm (or chilled, for that matter) without affecting your nutrient intake or wellness goals. The structure is important, the habit is important, the recipes are important, but otherwise there is a lot of flexibility so that you can make the soup cleanse experience yours. Nothing in this world is one size fits all!

And what if there's a particular category of soups that you really don't like? Here's how to substitute. If you don't like:

- Purees: Add another stew
- Beans: Add another stew
- Sweets: Add another puree or broth
- Stews: Add another puree or beans and lentils
- Broths: Add another puree

In the next few pages, I'll take you through five Soup Cleanse Plans (one from each health category). I'll also give you a calendar that shows my favorite soup regimens throughout the year, because I love to mix up my routine based on what is available at my farmers' market. You can follow these plans as I've laid them out, or you can head straight into the recipes to customize your own unique experience.

ENERGIZE

Energy is one of the biggest reasons many of us decide to change our diets. Feeling tired all the time really is the pits. These soups have a higher carbo-

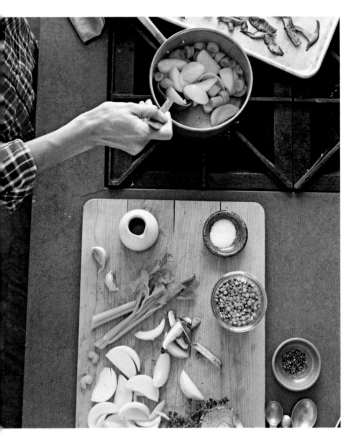

hydrate concentration than others because your body can use this fuel as energy more quickly than fat or protein. I know what you are thinking—carbs are bad! But complex carbohydrates from whole plants are not the enemy. Your body digests these carbohydrates in a more deliberate, even fashion than, say, a doughnut hole. A doughnut hole is a rapid, no-holds-barred, simple-carbohydrate (read: sugar) binge. Your body moves that fuel right to your bloodstream, and if it isn't used up by working muscles, it gets converted to fat stores. Complex carbohydrates are exactly what they sound like—they are more complicated, they have more going on. It takes a little longer for your body to pull out their carbohydrate fuel, and in the process, your body absorbs all the other gifts that those fruits and veggies have to offer, like antioxidants and vitamins and that beautiful thing called fiber. And those carbohydrates do indeed get used as energy for your body because they are released evenly—at a pace more familiar to your body, so you can use them rather than store them. The recipes in this category also have extra superfood ingredients that awaken the senses and stimulate the metabolism. Fresh and spicy ingredients like ginger, ground red pepper (cayenne), turmeric, mint, and lemon zest keep your senses alert.

Mix and match your favorite soups labeled as "Energize" to create your own plan, or try my favorite combination. I like it when my kids have to keep up with me, not the other way around. I can outpace even the most rambunctious toddler with this menu.

STRENGTHEN

For those of you who simply cannot function without challenging your muscles on a daily basis, this is a Soup Cleanse Plan that will keep you moving and fueled, even on your Soup Cleanse Day. I still recommend taking it easier than on a typical day, but, as always, pay attention to your body's cues and stay connected to avoid fatigue. Soups in this cleanse are more calorically dense and higher in protein than others. In fact, there are at least 8 grams of protein in every recipe here. This is a great regimen for those people who are on their feet all day or who know they have a stressful week ahead (critical thinking needs more energy, too). The body-loving fats in this regimen will help with satiety, as well.

I enjoy channeling my inner warrior every so often. If I'm feeling particularly driven by a workout buddy or just getting my groove on with a new high-intensity workout, then I like a little more oomph in my cleanse. I start the day with the creamy green pea soup, and then I feed my muscles with the Chickpea Stew, the Pear and Sunflower Seed soup, and the Antioxidant Stew. The White Miso with Peas and Thai Basil is the perfect post-workout soother for already aching muscles. Plus, I can sip it straight out of a mug if my arms are too shaky from all those triceps lifts. True story.

DETOX

Detox recipes are higher in fiber—hello, broom of the system, yes, we know what you do, and that's exactly what we're looking for! These recipes are also higher in electrolytes, which play a role in ensuring the filtration systems of the kidneys and liver work well. I call this the buff-and-shine because your body detoxifies already, and these soups just help the process work smoother and more efficiently.

I like this cleanse before and after big "dance around the fire" events. Celebrations like weddings, big birthdays, graduations—these call for a dance around the fire with the people closest to my heart. Sometimes that dance lasts more than a few days. I'm pretty balanced from souping over the past several years, and unlikely to saddle up to the open bar, but I'm apt to be hugging, laughing, and dancing until sunrise. And if someone pops open prosecco with the morning light, I'm likely to share in a toast. The Detox Cleanse is like my mom waking me up at 8 a.m. to make sure I make it to the Saturday track meet. Groggy and sluggish (and hungover) as I may be, she stands, toes tapping, at my bedroom door to make sure I'm moving. The Detox Cleanse wakes me up and moves the prosecco and 4 a.m. grilled cheese out of my system. This menu pushes me back toward my equilibrium in swift order. Or at least more swiftly than if I allowed myself to sleep in and order a bagel sandwich!

1. **Eggplant Tahini (page 65)**

2. **Green Chili (page 100)**

3. **Berry and Flaxseed (page 120)**

4. **Avocado Kimchi Stew (page 169)**

5. **Lemon-Fennel Consommé (page 183)**

WEIGHT LOSS

Higher-water-content vegetables tend to provide more volume without affecting calorie load. These soups are carefully selected so you start with a denser, more caloric soup and graduate to some of our lightest soups. Research shows that the philosophy of eating breakfast like a king, lunch like a prince, and dinner like a pauper holds true: By having your lighter soups at the end of the day, you are decreasing your risk of having leftover energy that won't be put to use before bedtime, and you train your body to enjoy heartier mornings. I also pick soups with higher satiety for the middle of the day because it's nothing but trouble to get to your 4 p.m. soup and think, I'm famished! *Deprivation* is a four-letter word. And while I don't love this philosophy, I do have clients who set up 2- or 3-day cleanses once a quarter to push their weight loss goals a little further. This is something you should explore with your physician, though, because it's a prolonged "lean" period. If it's done with the right preparation and the right mind-set, these additional Soup Cleanse Days can make a huge difference in both losing weight and gaining a deeper connection to eating habits and behaviors. Here's a lovely menu that I came up with after the birth of my first son, Grover. He was born in May and the ingredients in this soup reflect the new growth and warmth of that time of year. This is my spring weight loss cleanse.

1. **Creamy Gazpacho with Almonds (page 62)**

2. **Spring Favas with Asparagus, Lemon, and Dill (page 109)**

3. **Vanilla Pistachio with Oats (page 127)**

4. **Courgette Stew (page 144)**

5. **Daikon Radish with Tamarind and Spinach (page 173)**

And here's a menu inspired by my winter boy, Caleb, who was born December 7. This time of year can be trying for weight loss because our bodies crave the warmth and density that is generated by comfort foods. Traditional comfort foods are often high in starchy refined carbs and fats that are nutrient deficient. The soups in my winter weight loss cleanse create that comfort feel, but the carbs and fat are nutrient dense.

1. **Herbed Dairy-Free Cream of Mushroom (page 68)**

2. **Black Lentils with Coffee and Shiitakes (page 97)**

3. **Sweet Potato Soup with Persimmons and Pomegranate (page 135)**

4. **Potato and Cabbage Paprikash (page 166)**

5. **Cabbage Borscht (page 179)**

HEAL

Aren't all soups healing? Definitely, but some ingredients help your cells recover from damage and boost your body's natural repair cycle better than others. When we're recovering from sickness or surgery or battling chronic illness, we want our bodies to activate the anti-inflammatory response. Reducing inflammation isn't just about settling bloat or puffiness, although that's a good way to think about inflammation at a macro level. At a cellular level, inflammation is the body's natural ability to fend off intruders like harmful bacteria and viruses. The white blood cells swarm the intruder to prevent it from spreading. There's a balance with this system, though: We want it turned on just long enough to incapacitate the intruder. After that, we want it to be super chill, as if in a resting state. Unfortunately, the inflammatory response can be triggered when it's not needed, or it never chills out, and this causes us to feel sick and tired and to even experience chronic pain or depression. Arthritis, cancers, even Alzheimer's disease are thought to be closely linked to the inflammatory response. Unsurprisingly, a longstanding diet deficient in nutrient-rich whole foods—like plants, nuts, seeds, and whole grains—can also lead to chronic problems with inflammation.

This is why the menu for the Heal Cleanse focuses on ingredients that are rich sources of anti-inflammatory agents—the elements that help the inflammatory response stay in that chilled-out zone. All plants and vegetables have anti-inflammatory properties, but some are more powerful than others. Ingredients like turmeric, baby greens, mushrooms, and sprouted beans are key here. The golden child of the omega-3 fatty acid family is DHA, commonly found in marine sources like fatty cold-water fish (think wild salmon). DHA omega-3s have been shown to have powerful anti-inflammatory properties, and in addition to fish, they are found in algae, which is why I pick a few soups containing spirulina for this menu. Ingredients rich in ALA omega-3s—like flaxseed, pumpkin seeds, hempseed, and walnuts—are often touted for their healthful impact on the cardiovascular system, but they help tip your system toward that happy, anti-inflammatory state, as well. The Heal Cleanse menu:

1. Carrot and Turmeric (page 81)

2. Plant-Based Tagine (page 103)

3. Creamy Cocoa with Sweet Potatoes (page 121)

4. Summer or Fall Ratatouille (pages 150 and 153)

5. Ginger Broth with Napa Cabbage and Carrots (page 195)

what about all those nutrition facts?!

I'm a big believer in focusing more on the quality of ingredients and the ritual you create with your finished soups . . . and less on the numbers behind each recipe. The goal is always to reconnect with yourself so you can appreciate the good food you are creating, and sometimes the numbers on a label can get distracting and cause more anxiety than is necessary. With that said, it is important for some of us to pay careful attention to particular nutrition facts because of a medical condition or lifestyle choice. For this reason, we keep all the detailed nutrition facts listed on SplendidSpoon.com.

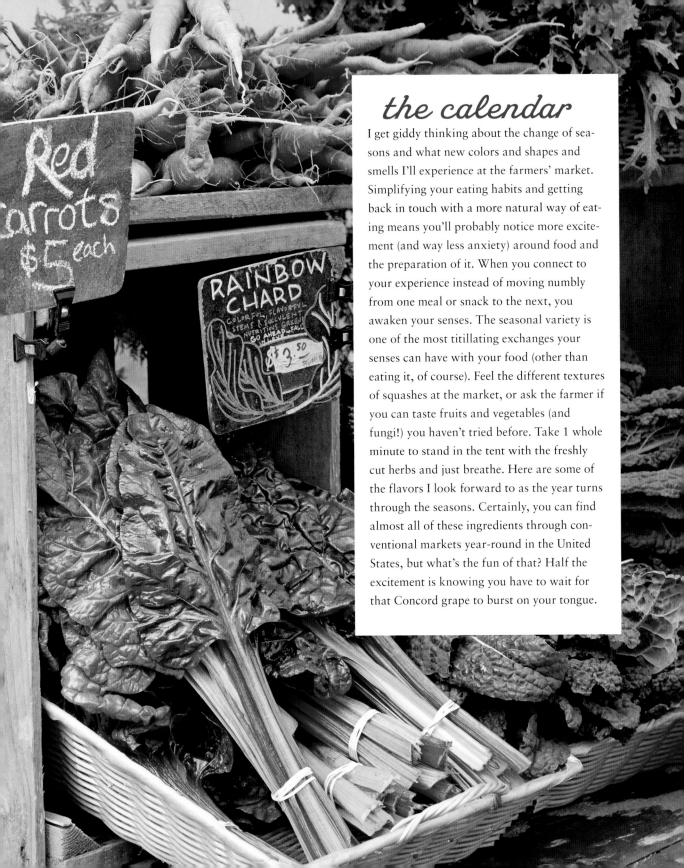

the calendar

I get giddy thinking about the change of seasons and what new colors and shapes and smells I'll experience at the farmers' market. Simplifying your eating habits and getting back in touch with a more natural way of eating means you'll probably notice more excitement (and way less anxiety) around food and the preparation of it. When you connect to your experience instead of moving numbly from one meal or snack to the next, you awaken your senses. The seasonal variety is one of the most titillating exchanges your senses can have with your food (other than eating it, of course). Feel the different textures of squashes at the market, or ask the farmer if you can taste fruits and vegetables (and fungi!) you haven't tried before. Take 1 whole minute to stand in the tent with the freshly cut herbs and just breathe. Here are some of the flavors I look forward to as the year turns through the seasons. Certainly, you can find almost all of these ingredients through conventional markets year-round in the United States, but what's the fun of that? Half the excitement is knowing you have to wait for that Concord grape to burst on your tongue.

JANUARY

Grapefruit and Fennel Consommé (page 128); Black Lentils with Coffee and Shiitakes (page 97)

FEBRUARY

Winter Root Vegetable Stew (page 147); Avocado Kimchi Stew (page 169) (This is because I'm really looking for some green as February comes to a close and the snow is still up to my hips. Avocado grows year-round in areas like California and Florida. If you're lucky to live in one of these areas, check out your local farmers' market, or if you're feeling ambitious, plant an avocado tree in your backyard! It's tough to eat entirely local in the climates that experience a true winter, so I am totally fine with some organic avocados even though they have traveled farther than is ideal.)

MARCH

Mung and Quinoa Congee (page 91) (in like a lion—we need comfort!); Confetti Pho (page 180) (out like a lamb—or at least a beautiful bright bowl to celebrate that the end of winter is around the corner)

APRIL

Green Coconut Curry with Broccoli (page 158) (Sometimes you can get broccoli and other cruciferous greens in April, as greenhouse farms will take advantage of the longer days.); Black Rice with Beets and Sesame Seeds (page 157)

MAY

Classic Filipino Sinigang (page 196); Vegan Bone Broth (page 174) (The first of the greens will start to arrive in spinach, green garlic, and bok choy; throw them all into this broth and buy extras to munch on raw. The first sniff of spring has arrived!)

JUNE

Simply Asparagus (page 70); Spring Favas with Asparagus, Lemon, and Dill (page 109)

JULY

Raw Native Corn with Basil (page 131); Raw Cashew and Cucumber (page 78)

AUGUST

Spiced Fig and Cashew (page 137) (Whenever the figs appear, snatch them and eat them raw, and then make this soup by the gallon and freeze it for the 11 months of the year the fig tree isn't bearing fruit.); Jalapeño Tomato Broth (page 187)

SEPTEMBER

Eggplant Tahini (page 65); Summer Ratatouille (page 150); Fall Ratatouille (page 153) (September is a miraculous month for vegetables, often providing traditional summer vegetables, like tomatoes and zucchini, right alongside fall vegetables, like butternut squash and Brussels sprouts.)

OCTOBER

"Chicken" Stew with Rice (page 161); Cranberry Beans and Kabocha Squash Stew (page 164) (The beauty of those first squashes can be as exciting as seeing those asparagus spears back in June. The changing seasons require our bodies to shift into a colder environment, and sometimes this happens very quickly. That jolt often brings coughs and sniffles, so I like making a big pot of comforting stew like "Chicken" Stew with Rice to bolster my defenses.)

NOVEMBER

Sweet Potato Soup with Persimmons and Pomegranate (page 135); Sunchoke and Celeriac with Parsley (page 57) (Isn't it fun when the produce matches your mood? I had to include persimmon and pomegranate here.)

DECEMBER

Roasted Chestnuts with Saigon Cinnamon (page 138); Potato and Cabbage Paprikash (page 166)

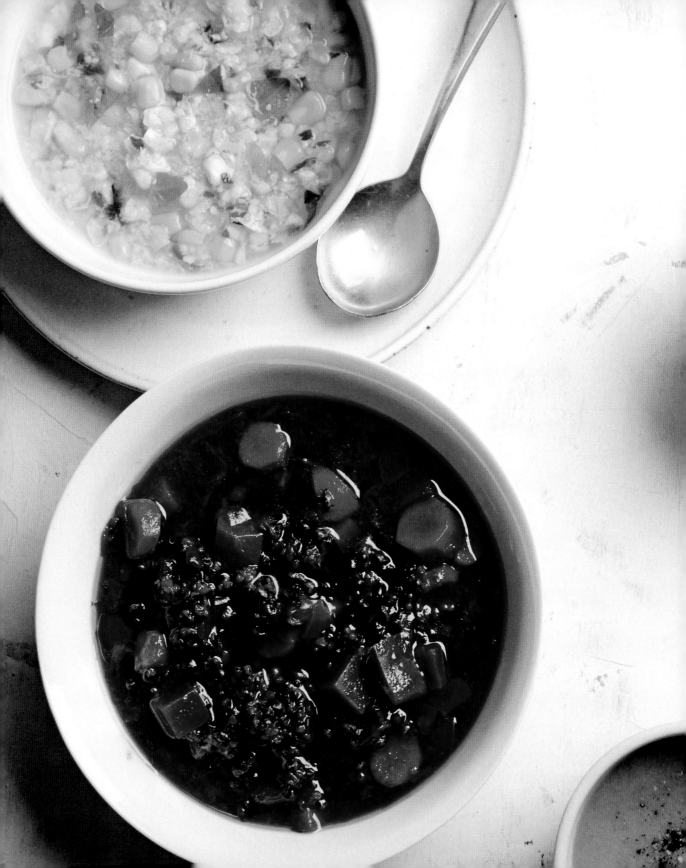

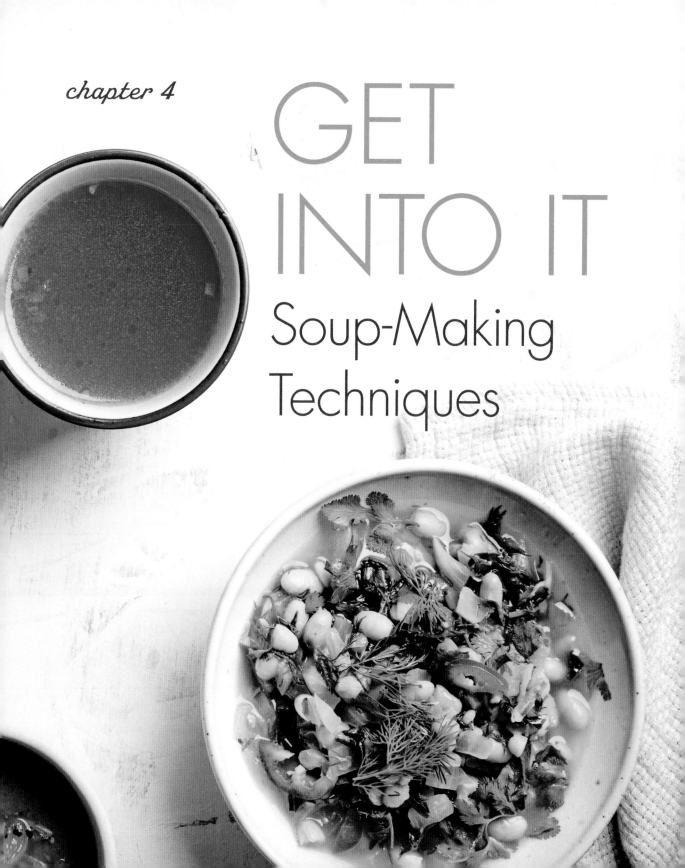

chapter 4

GET INTO IT

Soup-Making Techniques

ONE OF MY FAVORITE THINGS about soup is that it really is not very fancy. Sophisticated equipment and advanced kitchen experience are thankfully not necessary to create soups dense in both nutrition and flavor. Having said that, there are a handful of terms that I use throughout my recipes that have flexible interpretations depending on who you talk to. Here are my definitions for tools and techniques so we can start souping with a shared kitchen vocabulary.

The Tools

Forget all the shiny new tools. This is a book for the minimalist or the impatient, or both (like me). It's not even a requirement to make loads of broth for my soups. Water does just fine, and so do these tools. Here's what to dust off in your kitchen, starting with your trusty spoon.

- WOODEN SPOON. I've probably made 50 percent of these recipes with just a wooden spoon and a heavy-bottom pot. Wooden is my prefer-

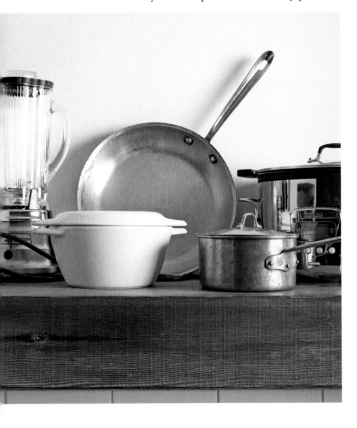

ence because you don't have to worry about scratching the bottom of your pot, and there's something really warm and genuine about a wooden spoon. This must be purely psychological, but a wooden spoon feels more like an extension of my hand than a metal one. I feel like it does what I want it to better than other materials. If you really like your metal spoon, then use it; your soup will probably come out better because you're more confident cooking with that metal spoon. Hey, whatever works.

- HEAVY-BOTTOM POT. This really makes a difference. Enameled cast-iron pots made by brands like Staub and Le Creuset disperse heat evenly, and they retain that heat so when you do things like turn off the stove and add spinach, the temperature remains consistent long enough to cook the spinach just right with the carryover heat.

- SKILLET. A skillet makes quicker work of getting aromatics to that soft and golden state of sweetness. It's also perfect for recipes like the Simply Asparagus (page 70), where you cook one vegetable (asparagus) a little differently than others (scallions and garlic).

- BAKING SHEET. Any cookie sheet will do. I cover mine in foil before roasting to make cleanup, well, cleaner (and quicker).

- LADLE. You could pour, but every soupie worth her weight in gold will want her own ladle.

- BLENDER OR IMMERSION (STICK) BLENDER. Almost all of us have a countertop blender that works really well for all recipes that need to be pureed. If you really want to go out and get a special tool to symbolize your newfound dedication to yourself through soup, I'd suggest an immersion (or stick) blender. This slender tool has a scary looking open blade at the bottom, but if you use it properly (the blade end immersed completely in the soup), you will want to use it for any recipe that calls for a puree. Immersing the blender in the soup means you won't have to ladle hot soup into a blender in batches, and cleanup is simpler with this little kitchen gadget.

- BOWLS FOR PREPARED INGREDIENTS. Organization is key. Have a stack ready to go and you won't get stuck with cutting board pileup. You'll thank me when you get to the Confetti Pho (page 180) or the Fall Ratatouille (page 153).

Knife Skills

Fancy knife work is totally unnecessary with the Soup Cleanse. Your cells don't know the difference between a chiffonade and a julienne, and you don't need to either. There are a handful of recipes, like the Confetti Pho and the Fall and Spring Ratatouilles, that ask for ribbons or small dice. Sure, it will make your soup look more beautiful if your ribbons are long and slender and your dice are uniform, but only do that kind of thing if you're really into presentation. I love making soups look beautiful because it makes me proud of my work in the kitchen and it elevates my experience when I eat—and I went to culinary school, so that's, like, my thing. But a lot of the time, I just go for the 'ish rule: skinny-ish carrots, cube-ish size and shape. The soup will still be perfectly delicious, and free form is totally eye-catching, too.

Cooking Temperatures

Put simply, you don't want to boil and you don't want to char. A simmer is gentle movement and little bubbles in your soup, a strong simmer is a little more movement, and boiling is when your soup is starting to jump out of the pot with a lot of movement and big bubbles. Simmer, that's great. Strong simmer, fine. Rolling boil, whoa, back off the flame a bit. I pick ingredients that have nutrient profiles that are relatively unaffected by heat, but when you hit a boiling point of 212°F, things start to break down. So just keep it at a simmer. When roasting, don't go over 425°F to prevent nutrient loss. You don't want to get a deep-black "burnt" char on your vegetables; burnt vegetables can contain small amounts of carcinogenic compounds. (You've probably heard a lot about carcinogens in burnt meat, which tend to be more concerning because they are more potent than in burnt veggies.) The point is to avoid a char so you can be confident your butternut squash is packing as much vitamin A as it can. Golden and dark brown is great—that's what gives your soup more nuanced flavor. Blackened is not great, and if it's not the nutrient factor that keeps you from enjoying that vegetable, the bitter taste of burn will.

Seasoning

At Splendid Spoon we strive to create soups that are as nutritious as they are spoon-licking good. I am not afraid of sea salt, or salt in general, for that matter. At the cellular level, ion channels are literally paramount to a functioning body—and sodium and potassium are what make these channels hum. They allow nutrients into our cells and push waste out. Too much salt can make you hold on to water, causing cells and blood vessels (and, yes, you) to bloat. This bloat can be really dangerous to someone predisposed to high blood pressure. However, most of the excessive salt in our diets comes from hidden salt lurking in packaged food (a lot of it is there to increase shelf life or to push flavor profiles into that heady pleasure zone). A full day of soup, selecting one from each category, will never exceed more than the RDI (Reference Daily Intake) of 2,300 milligrams. If you are sensitive to salt or eat a low-sodium diet for any reason at all, I suggest omitting salt from the recipes altogether and keeping a small salt cellar (a cute little saucer just right for two fingers to pinch a bit of brine) next to your soup. You'll add less salt at the moment of consumption because your palate will pick up on the little granules at the surface of your soup working their magic to help you perceive more flavors from the soup. Because good seasoning does that: You add just enough to enhance the other flavors. If you don't want to add salt at all, fresh herbs, lemon zest, and a squeeze of citrus are all great additions to create a more flavorful souping experience.

The Three Essential Elements of Souping

Here are the three elements I consider with every soup I make. Sooner than you think, you'll probably start experimenting with your own soup recipes, and this soup trine can be your key.

Chewing

Your digestive process starts in your mouth, and chewing is what gets things going. Moving your jaw and breaking down bits and pieces of food releases digestive enzymes in your mouth and sends signals to your stomach that something is coming. This part of the souping routine is important because it helps your body acknowledge that it is eating, and if you take your time chewing, you will feel full sooner because your stomach will be in sync with how much food you're taking in. If you gulp down your food quickly, not only will you miss out on the digestive enzymes in your mouth, but you also might swallow more air, which will contribute to gas. It will also take you a little longer to really perceive how full you are because food is rushing into your stomach before your stomach knows it's coming.

I keep lots of vegetable chunks in my broths, and I puree until smooth but rarely to a truly liquefied form. It would be tough, for example, to suck down all these soups with a straw. And that's the point: Bits of unpureed carrot and a little mushroom piece in your broth will remind you to chew. Chewing will help you slow down. It's all part of the soup helping you establish better habits.

Brightness

The body of a soup might be green, like Raw Cashew and Cucumber (page 78), Simply Asparagus (page 70), or Green Chili (page 100); or earthy, like Black Rice with Beets and Sesame Seeds (page 157) or Sunchoke and Celeriac with Parsley (page

57); or rich, like Potato and Cabbage Paprikash (page 166), or Creamy Cocoa with Sweet Potatoes (page 121), and they all benefit from brightness. Brightness often comes from an acid like vinegar or lemon juice that has just a prick of tart or sharp to offset the denser flavors of a soup. You can also add brightness with a fresh leafy herb like basil, mint, cilantro, or parsley. It is what separates a blah soup from a la-la-la-lovely soup. And if you ever end up with a blah soup, try saving it with a squeeze of lime or lemon or a sprinkle of mint or cilantro.

The Muse

This is a little harder to explain. The muse is the ingredient that inspires the rest of the recipe. It's usually the ingredient that is highest in volume after broth or water, and it's the one that you notice most in texture and taste. A lot of times the muse comes from a starchier ingredient—like the squash in the Cranberry Beans and Kabocha Squash Stew (page 164) or the sweet potato in the Cumin Sweet Potato

(page 58). Other times, it's a little more behind the scenes, like the tomato in the Fall Ratatouille (page 153); there are equal parts squash and kale and only a little bit more tomato, but it's the tomato's deep, sweet-tart taste that you perceive first. Another example of a behind-the-scenes muse is the navy beans in the Bell Pepper Bisque (page 94). With this soup, I notice the deliciously creamy texture first and then the sharper, vibrant flavor of the red bell peppers comes through.

The muse is like the host of a party. It's her smile that you notice first when you arrive, and she makes sure every newcomer is acknowledged, introduced, and comfortable. As soon as she leaves the room, something is missing. The muse is the main attraction that sparkles when combined with the sweetness of the onions and garlic, reflects bright citrus back onto your palate, and sets the tone for the overall mouthfeel of your soup. The soup would fall apart without the muse. Like the host of a party, she is there to help her guests open up and shine, but it's her personality that sets the tone.

That's a Big Pot
How to Store and Save Your Soup

Please read this before embarking on an epic weekend of soup-making. Every recipe in this book will give you four bowl-size portions. Therefore, five recipes will give you 20 portions, enough for 2 weeks of the 7-day Soup Cleanse. You can store each recipe in a large resealable container, or you can do what I do and portion each recipe into four containers so they are totally ready to eat when you are dashing out the door to work, or running home after a longer-than-usual day. You will need 20 quart-size bags or 20 plastic 16-ounce containers, a permanent marker, and some masking tape. Plastic 16-ounce containers actually fill closer to

18 ounces if you fill to the brim, so fill these containers with a half-inch of space from the top. Then make a label with the masking tape with the date, soup category, number (so you remember in which order you will be eating them), and soup name. If you are using plastic bags, make sure to store them flat in the freezer.

Soups will stay in great shape in your freezer for up to a month and in decent shape (meaning some of the flavor will diminish but nutrients will not) up to 3 months. Soups will stay in good shape in your fridge for a week, but nutrient loss is more rapid in the refrigerator because the temperature allows for oxidation. Oxidation is what happens as air mixes with your food and causes it to degrade. While most of these soups won't go bad after a week in the fridge, their nutrient profiles will shift downward. This is why I love freezing. It gives you more flexibility to eat the soups without worrying about nutrient loss. Plus, you have more flexibility with a frozen soup in transit; I can put a frozen container of Lentil and Kale (page 88) in my bag and not worry about it being out all day because the soup will stay fresh as it thaws slowly. Keep in mind that thaw time will be much faster in August than, say, November. Also, I suggest putting soups in a canvas bag before stowing in the same tote that your laptop goes in. Frozen soup does create condensation. Also, you don't want to end up with a purse full of black beans if the subway doors close on you and the plastic container pops open.

Gasp, plastic? If you're going to freeze, then you should store in plastic. I believe there are silicon and metal storage containers that would work, as well, but I eat *a lot* of soup, and I have always found these containers to be expensive, so I have yet to splurge. Let your soup cool in a big metal or glass bowl before pouring into the plastic, buy BPA-free containers, and do your best to pour your soup into a mug or bowl to reheat when you enjoy the soup later. It's not the best idea to freeze in glass because if you overfill, you could end up with shattered glass in your freezer. You can do it, though, and this is how. Use 24-ounce mason jars and fill with 2 inches remaining at the top. Place a label on the side of the glass (same as above) and store without a top. The topless jar will allow the soup to escape if you mistakenly overfill. Remember, the soup doesn't know if there's a top on it or not, so it could expand to the point of breaking your glass jar if you cover it tightly with a lid. It's not ideal to have lentils in the freezer, but it's definitely better than shards of glass. When you're ready to go, just take out your jar and screw a lid on.

Reheating

I am a huge proponent of establishing a souping ritual. Find a favorite mug or bowl, and pour your soup into it every time you eat. The visual cue of that dish might even act like a talisman for your wellness plan—reminding and encouraging you to stick with this simpler, cleaner way of eating. My absolute favorite way to reheat: Pour the soup into a small pot, bring it to a simmer, and then transfer it to my favorite mug and spoon or sip slowly. If you are storing your soup in glass or BPA-free plastic, you can also reheat it in the storage container in a microwave oven for 2 minutes. Take care when removing the soup from the microwave as these containers can be tricky to handle when hot. If you think you'll be nuking your soups a lot (which is *totally* fine from a nutrition perspective), go get yourself a nice mug or bowl to keep at your desk, darnit. You deserve to eat out of proper dishware. And, yes, use a real spoon. Ditch that plastic utensil stuff, and maybe bring a cloth napkin to the desk-dining experience. Class it up!

part 2

THE
SOUP
RECIPES

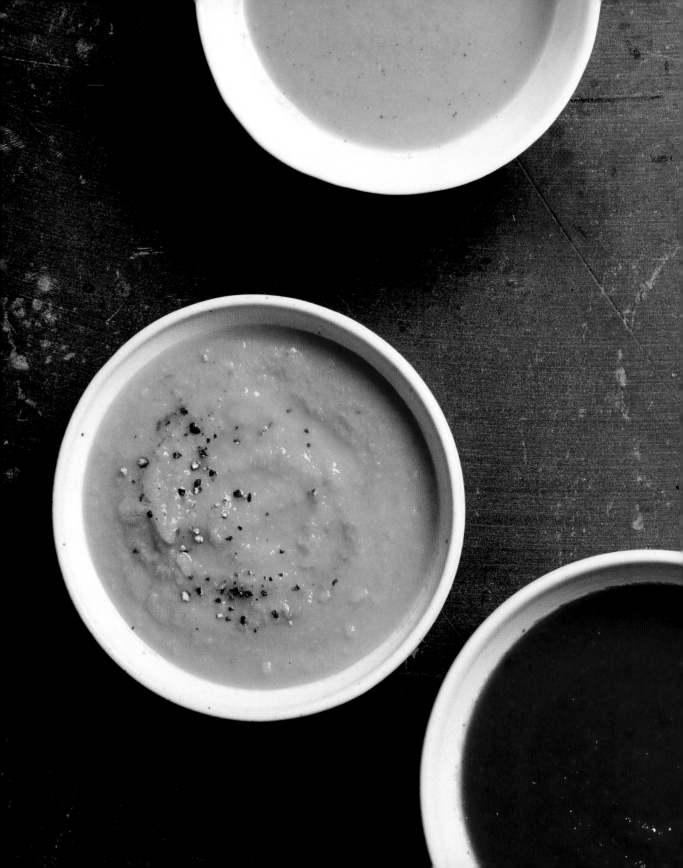

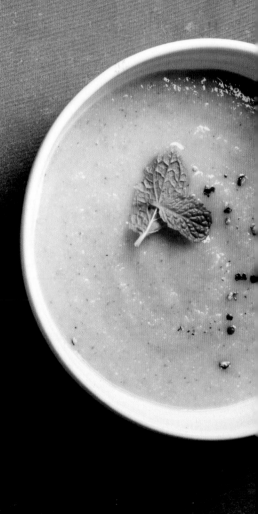

chapter 5

PUREES

at splendid spoon, we love purees. We bottle them up and drink them chilled on the go or heat them up for a super-comforting bisquelike experience. Pureeing begins the digestive process for you before the soup even hits your palate. This means the nutritional components are absorbed more quickly by the time they get into your gut. The other beautiful thing about purees is that your produce doesn't have to be so pretty. You won't notice bumps or bruises or other vegetal imperfections in your pureed soup, so why not go for some of the B-grade or "ugly" vegetables at the farmers' market (and thereby help lessen food waste)? You'll help the farmer monetize more of her crop, and you may even get a discounted price per pound. Like mama says, don't judge a book by its cover. It's what's inside that really counts!

I like starting the day with a puree, partly because the form is so perfect for rushed mornings. Of course, my favorite way to start the morning is with the newspaper laid out before me, a frothy Plant-Based Bulletproof Coffee (ahem, recipe on page 97), and my breakfast of choice on lovely white china. I read, sip, and savor at my own pace, which is usually over the course of 45 minutes. While I'd love to say I usually get to sit down and slowly spoon while sitting in front of the day's newspaper, it's more likely I'm putting together lunch boxes, cleaning up after my sons' breakfasts, packing a work bag, and just trying to enjoy the morning before I catapult myself out the door.

Pouring a just-warmed puree into a to-go coffee mug is often what saves me from a skipped breakfast. It feels like a slightly more sophisticated smoothie. It's savory, which reminds me that this is a meal, and it's warm, so I take my time to sip instead of drinking quickly to quench my thirst. I drink a big glass of room temperature water with lemon before and after I have my puree, which is my preferred form of hydration. This whole ritual (which happens over the course of 2 hours and is often interspersed with all the other things I do before 8 a.m.) starts two really important things. It activates my digestive system to begin fueling my already moving muscles, and it connects my intentions to my actions. I want to eat healthfully throughout the day, and here I am starting out with simple hydration and a pure, plant-based meal.

The simplicity and flexibility of purees, like those reliable-but-sometimes-too-sweet smoothies, make them a great choice for any mealtime that may be more rushed or frenzied. All my cleanse regimens start with a puree, but feel free to incorporate these recipes into the time of the day they will help you most.

SUNCHOKE *and* CELERIAC WITH PARSLEY

■ DETOX
■ HEAL

1½   pounds sunchokes, sliced

1½   pounds celeriac, peeled and sliced (save peel)

1   yellow onion, diced

1   clove garlic, minced

2   ribs celery, diced

2   tablespoons olive oil

2   quarts water

⅓   cup hazelnuts, soaked in water overnight and drained (see "Why Soak Your Nuts and Seeds?" on page 74 for more information)

1   teaspoon sea salt

Pinch of ground black pepper

Juice of ½ lemon

1   cup loosely packed and chopped fresh flat-leaf parsley

1. Preheat the oven to 425°F.

2. On a baking sheet, toss the sunchokes, celeriac, onion, garlic, and celery with the oil and spread into a single layer. Roast, stirring occasionally, for 25 minutes, or until the mixture is soft and very aromatic.

3. Meanwhile, in a pot over medium-high heat, bring the water to a simmer. Add the celeriac peel and any other vegetable trimmings you may have and simmer for 20 minutes.

4. Strain the vegetable trimmings out of the stock and pour half of the stock into a countertop blender. Add the roasted celeriac and sunchoke mixture, hazelnuts, salt, pepper, and lemon juice. Puree until very smooth with the lid vented, adding more stock as necessary to create a thin milkshake consistency. Add the parsley and puree.

5. Pour into warm bowls and enjoy.

Sunchokes are funny little root vegetables, also known as Jerusalem artichokes. They are available in the fall in the Northeast and in the winter months of warmer climates. I skip peeling because their skin is thin, there are nutrients in the skin, and they are funny shaped little buggers that defy every peeler I've ever owned. Sunchokes have a nutty texture and, although they are often fried up and roasted like potatoes, they aren't as starchy. I like complementing their nuttiness with hazelnuts, which also give the soup a creamier texture, and adding some brightness with celeriac and parsley.

some people avoid sunchokes like the plague because they contain inulin, which is a type of fiber that some people are very sensitive to. Read: It causes a lot of gas, cramping, and bloating. If this is you, but this soup sounds super yummy, sub the sunchokes with peeled and diced jicama. Add the jicama at the end (raw) just before blending since it doesn't need to be roasted.

CUMIN SWEET POTATO

1½ pounds sweet potatoes, peeled and cut into 1" chunks

¼ cup (about a handful) raw unsalted cashews, soaked in water overnight (see "Why Soak Your Nuts and Seeds?" on page 74 for more information)

½ cup loosely packed fresh cilantro

Pinch of ground red pepper

½ teaspoon ground cumin

½ teaspoon sea salt

4 cups water

1. Preheat the oven to 425°F.

2. Wrap the sweet potatoes in foil and place on a baking sheet. Bake for 25 minutes, or until a knife can be inserted and removed from the potatoes with ease. When the potatoes are done, open the foil carefully and let cool before handling.

3. In a countertop blender, combine the cooked potatoes, cashews and soaking water, cilantro, ground red pepper, cumin, salt, and 3 cups of the water. Blend until very smooth (you want a thin milk-shake consistency), adding the remaining water as needed to reach this consistency. Enjoy warm or chilled.

Note: You can roast the sweet potatoes whole, but they will take longer to cook.

I love this soup mainly because the rich texture feels and tastes much more decadent than it is but also because the fat from the cashews helps increase absorption of beta-carotene from the sweet potatoes. Beta-carotene is lauded for sharpening eyesight, and it's a key player in a healthy immune system. The ground red pepper and fresh cilantro add just the right amount of kick and freshness to excite your palate.

sweet potatoes and yams are tuberous root vegetables that come from a flowering plant, but when it comes to flavor, the sweet potato reigns supreme. Its flesh can be orange, white, yellow, or reddish and has a sweeter and more delicate flavor than the starchier yam. How to stay on point in the grocery aisle? Look for tapered ends and you'll always end up with the preferred sweet potato.

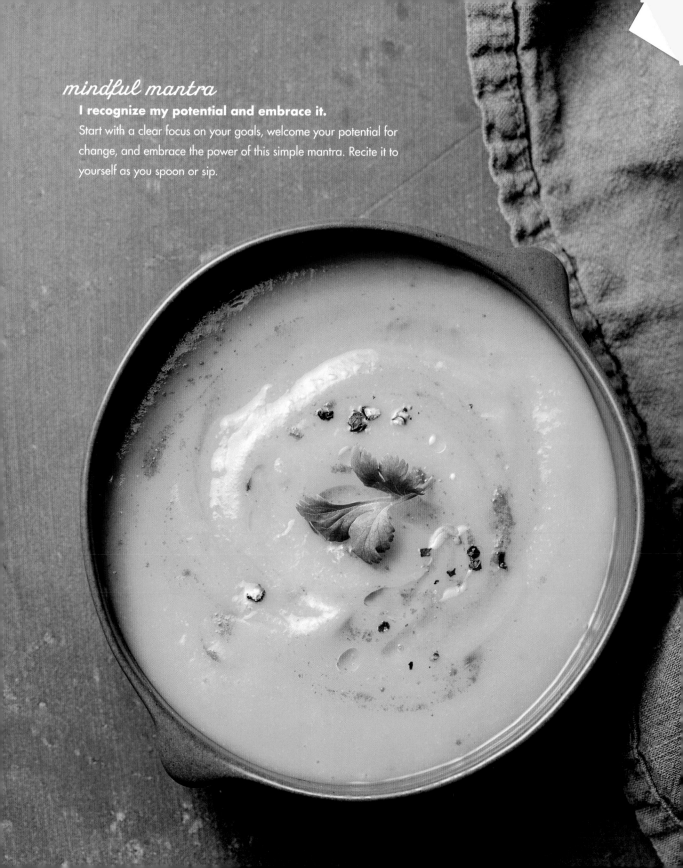

mindful mantra

I recognize my potential and embrace it.

Start with a clear focus on your goals, welcome your potential for change, and embrace the power of this simple mantra. Recite it to yourself as you spoon or sip.

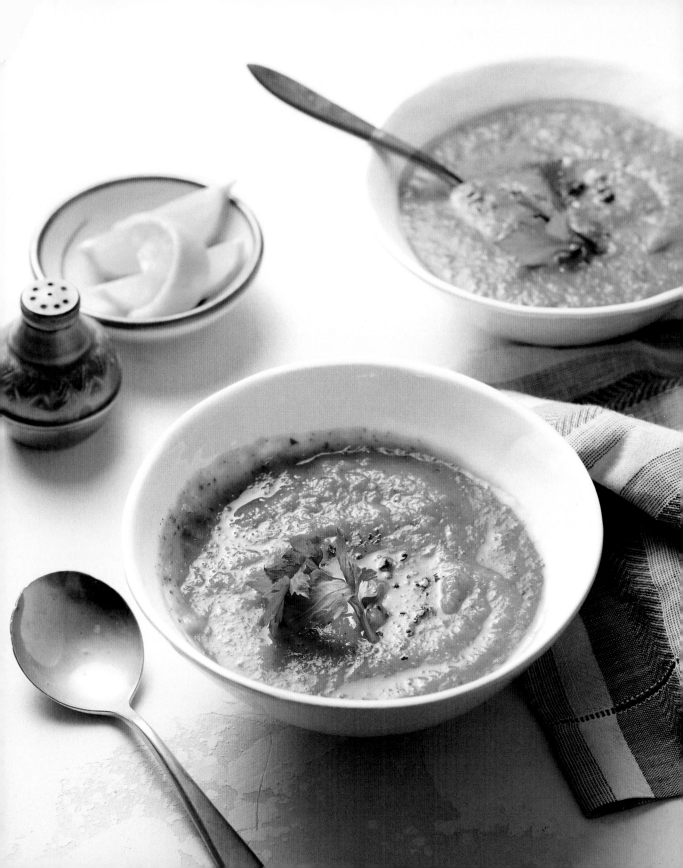

SPRING ALLIUM

2 tablespoons olive oil

1 bunch leeks, white part only, finely sliced

1 bunch scallions, white and green parts, sliced

1 bunch ramps or chives, chopped

1 pound celery, tops removed and thinly sliced

1 quart water plus more as needed

1 small white potato, diced

1 teaspoon finely chopped fresh thyme

1 teaspoon sea salt

Pinch of ground black pepper

Juice of ½ lemon

1. In a large pot over medium-high heat, warm the oil. Cook the leeks, scallions, ramps or chives, and celery for 5 to 10 minutes, or until soft and golden. Reduce the heat to low and cook for 20 minutes, or until the mixture is extremely soft and translucent (you want it to almost melt on the bottom of the pot). Add some of the water as needed to prevent the mixture from getting too dark and sticking to the bottom of the pot.

2. Add the potato, thyme, salt, pepper, and the remaining 1 quart water. Stir to combine and simmer for about 20 minutes to allow the flavors to meld.

3. Using an immersion blender or countertop blender, puree the soup until very smooth, adding more water as needed.

4. Add the lemon juice before serving. Enjoy warm or chilled.

HOW TO CLEAN AND PREP LEEKS

Remove the dark outer green part, and then slice off the dark green tip down where the leaf lightens to a pale green. Slice the stalk lengthwise, and then cut into the desired pieces. Rinse and strain.

■ ENERGIZE
■ WEIGHT LOSS

With starchy potato and a beautiful combination of leeks, scallions, and ramps, this puree is smooth and savory. There aren't any common yellow or red onions in this recipe at all! Instead, I picked vegetables from the onion family, alliums, that have a slightly greener, fresher, less pungent flavor. Leeks are delicate and creamy and traditional with potatoes, scallions are a little sharper and closer to that strong onion taste but with a flavor that stays lively even after cooking, and ramps—oh, ramps. Ramps are a special springtime-only treat. They look a lot like scallions but with wider leaves and a trademark stain of ruby on their white necks. They have a delicate onion flavor that kind of punches you with pepper after a few seconds of chewing. You can smell the peppery-ness if you hold a bunch to your nose at the farmers' market. That's my idea of a perfect bouquet. I'll take an armful of ramps over a bunch of daffodils any spring day.

CREAMY GAZPACHO
with ALMONDS

2 tablespoons olive oil

2 pounds tomatoes (any variety), diced (seeded or unseeded is fine)

1 cucumber, peeled, seeded, and chopped

2 scallions, chopped

1 bell pepper (any color), chopped

1 small jalapeño pepper, finely chopped (use gloves if your skin is sensitive to hot peppers)

1 quart water

½ teaspoon ground cumin

½ teaspoon sea salt

¼ cup raw unsalted almonds, soaked in water overnight and drained (see "Why Soak Your Nuts and Seeds?" on page 74 for more information)

½ cup loosely packed fresh basil, chopped

Any Spaniard would take issue with this being called gazpacho. Technically, gazpacho is a raw, chilled soup, and it can be made with just about any vegetable so long as it remains raw and chilled. Trouble is, tomatoes need some heat to really concentrate the antioxidant lycopene. A little time on the burner is all your gazpacho needs to amp up the lycopene quotient. The olive oil is key, too; as a fat-soluble nutrient, lycopene glides into your cells surrounded by this heart-healthy fat.

1. In a large pot over medium-high heat, warm the oil. Add the tomatoes, cucumber, scallions, bell pepper, and jalapeño pepper and stir. Cook for 15 minutes, or until the tomatoes break apart and the mixture becomes soft. Add some of the water if the mixture starts to stick to the bottom of the pot.

2. Stir in the remaining water, cumin, salt, and almonds, cover, and simmer for 10 minutes. At the last minute, toss in the basil.

3. Using an immersion blender or countertop blender, puree the soup until very smooth. Enjoy chilled for a more, dare I say, authentic gazpacho experience. Since the soup is cooked you're more than welcome to enjoy it warm, too (just call it tomato soup). And don't serve it as gazpacho to your Spanish friends.

THE SPICE TEST
Remember to taste the jalapeño pepper before adding it to the pot! Simply slice a tiny piece and touch the cut part to your tongue. Give it a minute for the hot oils to kick in. These peppers can vary wildly in spiciness, with some barely packing a punch and others delivering a wallop. Use more or less depending on your affinity for heat.

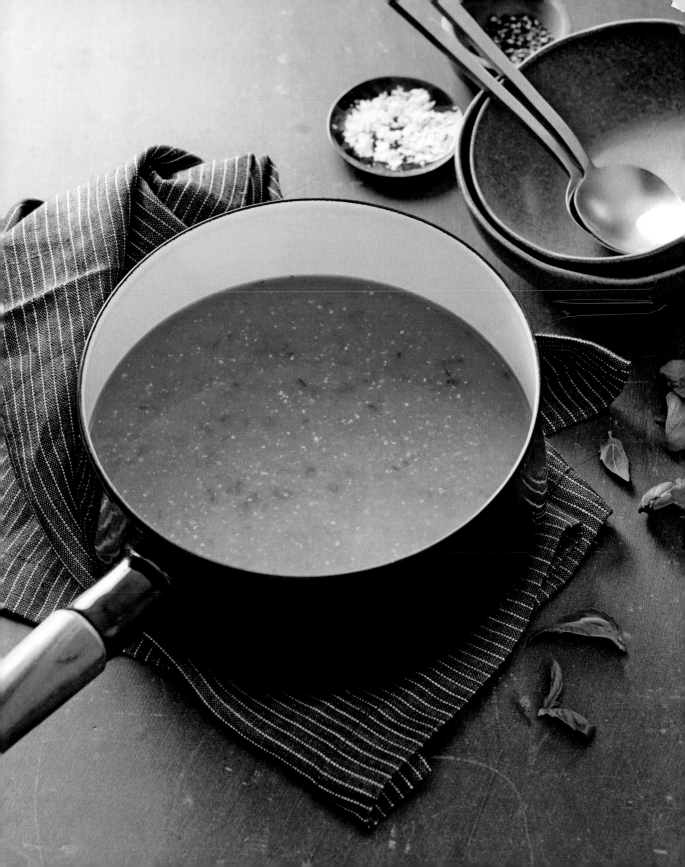

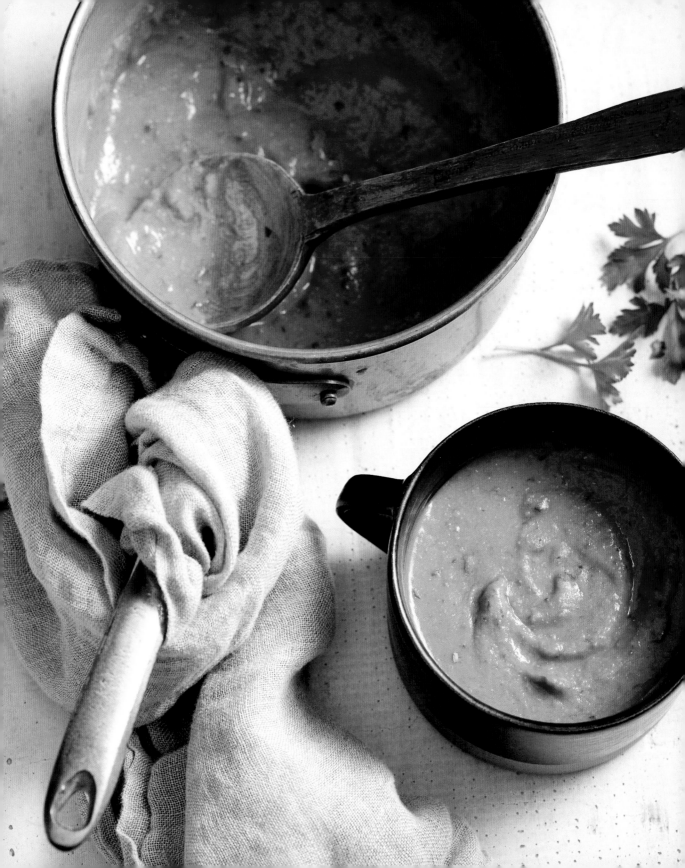

EGGPLANT TAHINI

1   large eggplant, diced (about 6 cups)

1   tablespoon olive oil

1   bell pepper (any color), diced

1   small onion, diced

1   clove garlic, minced

1   quart water

½   teaspoon ground cumin

½   teaspoon sea salt

1   tablespoon tahini (see note)

1   tablespoon chopped fresh flat-leaf parsley

    Peel of 1 lemon, grated (about 2 teaspoons)

1. Sprinkle the eggplant with a few pinches of salt and toss to coat. Set aside for 20 minutes.

2. Place the eggplant in a colander, rinse off the salt and bitter juices, and pat dry.

3. In a large pot over medium-high heat, warm the oil. Add the eggplant, pepper, onion, and garlic and cook for 5 minutes, stirring frequently, or until the vegetables are softened and browned. Reduce the heat to low and cook for 25 minutes, or until the mixture becomes very soft. Add some of the water if the mixture starts to stick to the bottom of the pot.

4. Stir in the cumin, salt, tahini, and the remaining water and simmer for 10 minutes. At the last minute, toss in the parsley and lemon peel.

5. Using an immersion blender or countertop blender, puree the soup until very smooth. Enjoy warm or chilled.

Note: If you can't find tahini, a Middle Eastern sesame paste, you can substitute with unsalted, unsweetened peanut butter.

I rented cooking space in a pizza restaurant in Greenpoint, Brooklyn, during its pre-pizza hours and cooked my first soups next to a pizza oven that was still ripping hot from the previous night's service. There was one morning when I had been overzealous with my heirloom eggplant haul at the farmers' market. I was staring at a pile of the little oblong beauties wondering what kind of soup was made exclusively with eggplant. As sweat streamed down my face, I remembered that eggplant was loaded with a unique combination of electrolytes—just what my body craved on a hot day. I piled my haul into the pizza oven, and then pureed them with tahini to create a baba ghanoush–inspired soup. Poured into a glass over ice, it was the perfect pick-me-up.

eggplant belongs to the nightshade family of vegetables, which also includes tomatoes, bell peppers, and potatoes. Technically, eggplant is the fruit of the plant, and it makes the perfect addition to vegetable soup. I don't recommend eating eggplants raw; it's a pretty unpleasant experience. Cooking transforms the flesh from a spongy mass into a silky-soft mush and mellows its intense, bitter flavor. It's best to slice your eggplant and sprinkle with salt to pull some of the bitter juices out of the vegetable's flesh. Rinse before cooking, and use plenty of heart-healthy fats to accelerate your body's access to the electrolytes in eggplant.

BUTTERNUT TURMERIC

1 butternut squash, quartered and seeded

2 tablespoons olive oil, divided

½ teaspoon sea salt

½ teaspoon ground black pepper

1 onion, diced

1 clove garlic, minced

1 rib celery, diced

1 tablespoon grated fresh turmeric (use a Microplane or the finest grade on a box grater) or 1 teaspoon dried

1 sprig fresh rosemary, woody stems removed and leaves finely chopped, or ½ teaspoon dried

1 teaspoon ground cinnamon

Freshly grated nutmeg, to taste

5 cups water

1. Preheat the oven to 425°F.

2. Rub the flesh of the squash with 1 tablespoon of the oil and season with the salt and pepper. Place the squash, flesh side up, on a baking sheet. Bake for 35 minutes, or until a knife can be inserted and removed from the squash with ease.

3. Meanwhile, in a medium pot over medium heat, warm the remaining 1 tablespoon oil. Cook the onion, garlic, and celery, stirring frequently, for 5 to 7 minutes, or until the vegetables are very soft and translucent. Add the turmeric, rosemary, cinnamon, and nutmeg and cook for 2 minutes, or until fragrant. Set aside.

4. Remove the squash from the oven and cool for 15 minutes. Scoop out the flesh with a spoon and discard the skins.

5. Add the squash flesh and water to the pot. Increase the heat to high to quickly bring the soup to a simmer. Reduce the heat to medium and simmer for 10 minutes.

6. Using an immersion blender, puree the soup until smooth. Enjoy warm.

■ HEAL
■ DETOX

Smooth and buttery, this golden squash lives up to its name, lending its smooth, autumnal flavor to this soup. Turmeric's bright, lightly sulfuric flavors possess anti-inflammatory components that are locked in the compound curcumin. Black pepper and heat are the keys that release its powers. This soup will fill your kitchen with an intoxicating aroma that may linger for a few days. Enjoy it! Studies show the scent of cinnamon releases endorphins. Smiling while spooning will absolutely improve your experience with this (and every) soup!

DRIED OR FRESH?
Dried herbs tend to do best if they're added *during* cooking so their flavors have time to infuse the whole dish, but fresh herbs are a little more flexible and can be used during or after. If you are omitting salt from the recipe for health reasons, add the fresh herbs at the end, or add an additional sprinkle of fresh herbs when you sit down to enjoy your soup.

If you're making a recipe that calls for fresh and you'd like to use dried—or vice versa— here's a general rule of thumb: If a recipe calls for fresh and you have dry, use half the volume. If it's the reverse, use twice the volume called for.

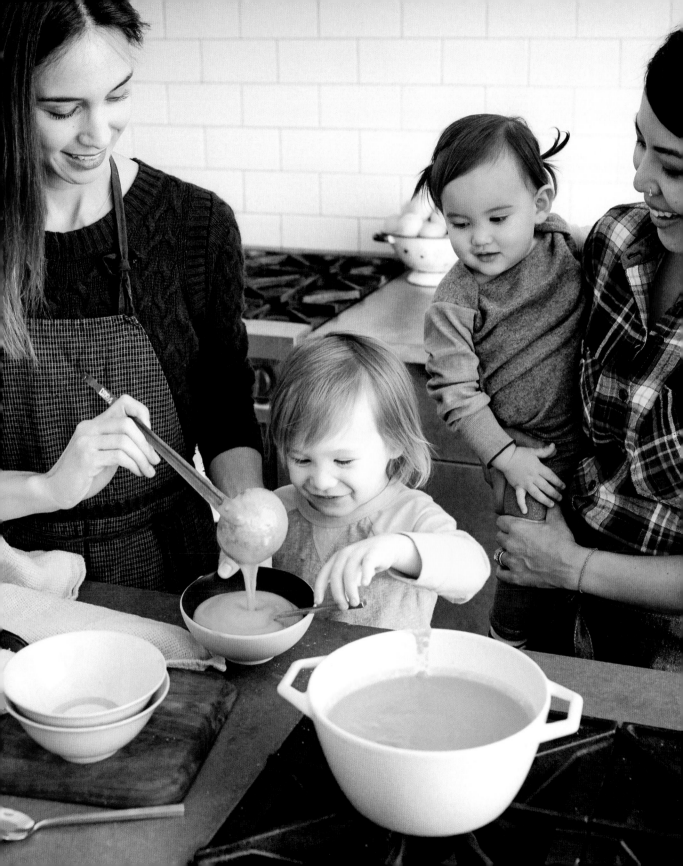

HERBED DAIRY-FREE CREAM OF MUSHROOM

2 pounds mixed shiitake and maitake mushrooms, stems removed and saved and tops roughly chopped

1 yellow onion, diced

1 clove garlic, chopped

2 ribs celery, diced

¼ cup coconut oil, melted

1 quart water

1 tablespoon chopped fresh dill (stems saved)

1 cup loosely packed fresh flat-leaf parsley (stems saved)

⅓ cup hazelnuts, soaked in water overnight and drained (see "Why Soak Your Nuts and Seeds?" on page 74 for more information)

¼ teaspoon ground black pepper

½ teaspoon sea salt

Juice of ½ lemon

1. Preheat the oven to 425°F.

2. Using your hands, coat the mushrooms, onion, garlic, and celery with the coconut oil. Place the vegetables on a baking sheet and roast, stirring occasionally, for 25 minutes, or until the mixture is soft and very aromatic.

3. Meanwhile, in a medium pot over medium-high heat, bring the water to a simmer. Add the mushroom stems, herb stems, and any other vegetable trimmings you may have. Cover and cook for 20 minutes.

4. Strain the vegetable trimmings out of the stock and pour into a counter-top blender. Add the roasted mushroom mixture, hazelnuts, dill, parsley, pepper, salt, and lemon juice. Puree until very smooth with the lid vented.

5. Pour into warm bowls and enjoy.

■ STRENGTHEN
■ MOM AND BABY
■ HEAL
■ WEIGHT LOSS

Trust me when I say this cream of mushroom soup will leave you in awe, wondering how you've managed to survive this long without enjoying hazelnuts in your soup.

BROTH ALERT: KEEP YOUR STEMS!

Have any mushroom stems, parsley stems, dill stems, or other stems or vegetable ends lying around? Save them for any of the broth recipes in Chapter 9. You can also wrap them up in a little sachet and add them to any recipe to infuse more vegetal flavor into your soup as it cooks. Simply wrap the veggie pieces and stems in a piece of cheesecloth, tie the ends closed with butcher's twine to create a sachet, and toss into any soup recipe for an extra layer of flavor. Remember to remove your sachet before pureeing or serving.

hazelnuts are sweet little edible kernels from the birch, or *Betulaceae,* family of trees. They are a rich source of potassium, calcium, copper, iron, magnesium, phosphorus, zinc, and selenium. These are minerals that the body uses for everything from basic cellular function (potassium) to bone health (calcium, magnesium, iron, and phosphorus) to metabolism (selenium) to immunity (zinc) and heart health (copper). Really, these minerals do lots of things for lots of parts of your body, but your body doesn't synthesize them, so go for more hazelnuts!

WHITE TURNIP *with* TURNIP GREENS

2 tablespoons olive oil

1 small yellow onion, diced

2 ribs celery, diced

1 cup white button mushrooms, diced

½ teaspoon sea salt

2 sprigs fresh thyme, woody stems removed and leaves finely chopped (see notes)

Pinch of ground black pepper

1 bunch turnips or 1 large turnip, white bulbs quartered and leafy green tops removed and chopped (see notes)

1 quart water

1. In a medium pot over medium heat, warm the oil. Cook the onion and celery, stirring frequently, for 5 to 7 minutes, or until the vegetables are translucent. Add the mushrooms, salt, thyme, and pepper and cook for 10 minutes, or until the mushrooms are very soft. Add the turnip greens and cook for 5 minutes. Remove some of the mixture and set aside as garnish.

2. Increase the heat to medium-high, add the water and turnip bulbs, and simmer for 15 minutes, or until the turnips are soft.

3. Using an immersion blender, puree the mixture until very smooth. Ladle the soup into warm bowls and garnish with the turnip green mixture.

Notes: When you are selecting turnips, go for the small white variety that look like radishes. These flaunt a sweeter and more delicate flavor than some of the larger turnips, commonly known as rutabagas.

Thyme has a long history of use in natural medicine in connection with chest and respiratory problems, including coughs, bronchitis, and congestion. The volatile oil components of thyme have also been shown to have antimicrobial activity against a host of different bacteria.

■ DETOX
■ WEIGHT LOSS

I am a member of a CSA (community supported agriculture program), which provides me with a share of the weekly harvest from a local farm. It's a fantastic way to sample whatever is growing while helping a farm offset its overhead because you pay for the share at the start of the growing season. The catch is, I don't get to choose my fruits and veggies each week, and lesser-known produce ends up in what's called a "swap box." Turnips always end up in the swap box. I felt that there must be something we were all missing with these turnips, and I was determined to find it. With their delicate flavor and beautiful white texture, turnips produce a really lovely soup. Their sometimes biting flavor is softened significantly in the cooking process. Sautéed mushrooms, with their delicate taste and texture, draw even more attention to that softened turnip flavor. And the totally edible, don't-throw-'em-out turnip greens add a shock of color to this otherwise muted soup—telling the spooner that, yes, there's more than meets the eye with turnips. Don't give up on them until you've dipped your spoon.

SIMPLY ASPARAGUS

■ MOM AND BABY
■ HEAL
■ DETOX

1 quart water

4 pounds fresh asparagus (see "Bend and Snap" for processing directions)

2 tablespoons olive oil

1 bunch scallions, chopped

2 ribs celery, sliced

2 sprigs fresh rosemary, woody stems removed and leaves finely chopped, or pinch of dried

Pinch of ground black pepper

1 teaspoon sea salt

1 quart ice cubes

Juice of 1 lemon

Asparagus holds its own with this fresh, green puree that's rich in flavor. Light notes of rosemary give it an herbal touch, while a zesty splash of lemon juice finishes the palate with a clean, acidic jolt.

1. In a large pot over high heat, bring the water to a boil while you prepare the asparagus. Add the woody asparagus ends to the boiling water, cover, reduce the heat to low, and simmer for 15 minutes.

2. Meanwhile, in a skillet over medium heat, warm the oil. Cook the scallions, celery, rosemary, and pepper, stirring frequently, for 5 to 7 minutes, or until the vegetables are soft. Set aside.

3. Remove the woody asparagus ends from the stock and discard or compost. Increase the heat to high and bring the stock back to a boil. Add the asparagus spears and salt and cook for about 10 minutes.

4. In a countertop blender, combine the ice, asparagus and stock, scallion mixture, and lemon juice. Blend until very smooth with the lid vented.

5. Pour into bowls and chill in the fridge for about 15 minutes before enjoying.

BEND AND SNAP

To determine the appropriate spot to trim your asparagus spears, simply grasp one spear on each end and bend until it snaps. Place the woody end in a bowl and the pretty pointed spear next to your remaining pile of untrimmed asparagus. Slice the remaining asparagus at the same place and keep all woody ends in a bowl for your asparagus stock. The spears will go into the body of your soup.

asparagus is a rich source of folate, which is critical to nervous system function. In fact, all women of "childbearing age" are told to consume significant quantities of folate before becoming pregnant as it significantly decreases the chances of neural tube defects in fetuses. Folate also contributes to the potential antiaging properties of this delicious spring veggie: It may help our brains fight cognitive decline.

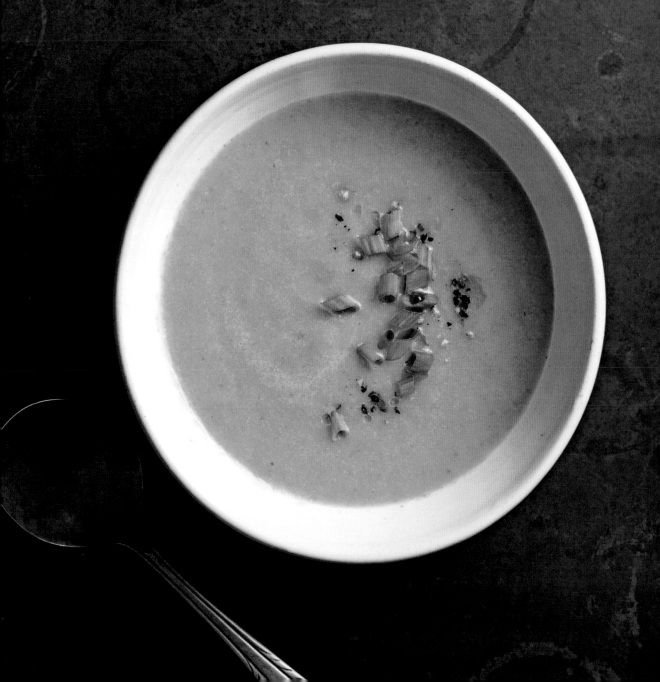

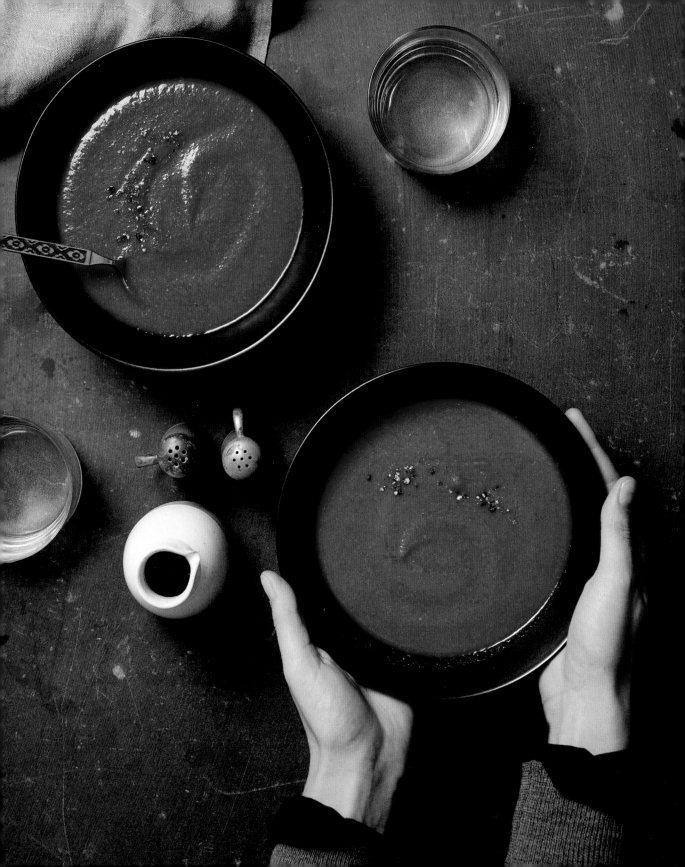

BEET BALSAMIC BISQUE

■ ENERGIZE
■ DETOX
■ HEAL

Beautiful beets are packed with detoxifying phytonutrients that fight inflammation as well as a flavor that's both sweet and earthy. This soup is mostly beets, which lets their flavor really stand out and keeps the recipe straightforward, making this soup a simple classic. Olive oil supports cardiovascular health and smooths out the texture to make it bisquelike.

3 large beets, quartered

1 tablespoon olive oil

1 large carrot, cut into small dice

1 small yellow onion, diced

1 clove garlic, minced

2 tablespoons chopped fresh dill

1 tablespoon grated fresh horseradish root (use a Microplane or the finest grade on a box grater) or prepared horseradish

1 teaspoon sea salt

Pinch of ground black pepper

1 quart water

1 tablespoon balsamic vinegar

1. Preheat the oven to 425°F.

2. Wrap the beets in foil and roast for 45 minutes, or until a knife can be inserted and removed from the beets with ease.

3. Meanwhile, in a medium pot over medium heat, warm the oil. Cook the carrot, onion, and garlic, stirring frequently, for 10 minutes, or until the vegetables are soft and sweet. Set the mixture aside while the beets continue to cook.

4. Remove the beets from the oven and let cool. Peel the skin from the beets and compost or discard the skin. (Don't spend too much time on this task if the peels are stubborn; a few bits and pieces won't affect the taste of your soup.)

5. In the same medium pot over medium heat, combine the beets with the carrot mixture. Add the dill, horseradish, salt, pepper, water, and vinegar and simmer for 15 minutes.

6. Using an immersion blender or countertop blender, puree the soup until very smooth. This soup is fantastic as a chilled soup-drink on the go or warm in a bowl.

drinking beetroot juice increases bloodflow to the brain (and everywhere else), so this soup may help you with stamina in the library, the gym, and well—the bedroom. Get it, girl.

CREAMY CAULIFLOWER
and LEEK

■ DETOX
■ HEAL
■ MOM AND BABY

¼ cup almonds, soaked in water overnight and drained (see "Why Soak Your Nuts and Seeds?" for more information)

1 small leek, white part only, or 1 bunch scallions, white and green parts, chopped

1 small head cauliflower, chopped into very small pieces (about 4 cups)

¼ cup apple cider vinegar

⅓ cup loosely packed fresh dill

½ teaspoon sea salt

Pinch of red-pepper flakes

2½ tablespoons olive oil

4 cups boiled water

1. In a countertop blender, combine the almonds, leek or scallions, cauliflower, vinegar, dill, salt, red-pepper flakes, oil, and water and cover tightly. Allow the mixture to sit for 20 to 25 minutes so the hot water cooks the cauliflower.

2. Vent the blender to release any steam, cover, and blend until very smooth. Add some cold water if necessary to achieve a milk-shake consistency.

3. Place in the refrigerator for 1 hour to chill before enjoying. The soup will cool faster if you portion it into separate containers. This soup is totally yummy warm, too!

WHY SOAK YOUR NUTS AND SEEDS?

Don't let their stationary state fool you—those nuts are alive! Nuts are actually the fruit of a plant, protecting a seed within them. Soaking nuts and seeds in water overnight activates lots of good enzymes that encourage the seed to germinate. Soaking also removes the protective, slightly toxic elements that prevent the seed from germinating until the correct (moist) conditions are met. Drain the soaking liquid before using the nuts. If you're really in a rush, you can soak them in boiled water for 30 minutes instead of overnight, but this is more for achieving the softer texture you want for the soup to blend nicely than for health reasons.

Cauliflower is one of those funny vegetables that everyone assumes isn't so great for you because of its color (or lack thereof). But remember when you looked at the color wheel in art class and your teacher told you that white is actually a mixture of all the colors—and it blew your mind?! Well, it blew my mind at least. Think of cauliflower in this same way. Sure we associate white food with refined things like white flour and sugars, but in nature white is still a color that signifies powerful phytochemical properties. Cauliflower is a cruciferous vegetable like broccoli, Brussels sprouts, and kale, the straight-A students sitting in the front row of veggie school. This means cauliflower has sulfur compounds that have been shown to fight off cancer cells and improve blood pressure and kidney function. Plus, cauliflower is really versatile in recipes: It can hold together as chunky florets or blend seamlessly into a puree, as it does here. So, yeah, don't get too comfortable with that 4.0 GPA kale, because cauliflower just may steal its place on stage as valedictorian.

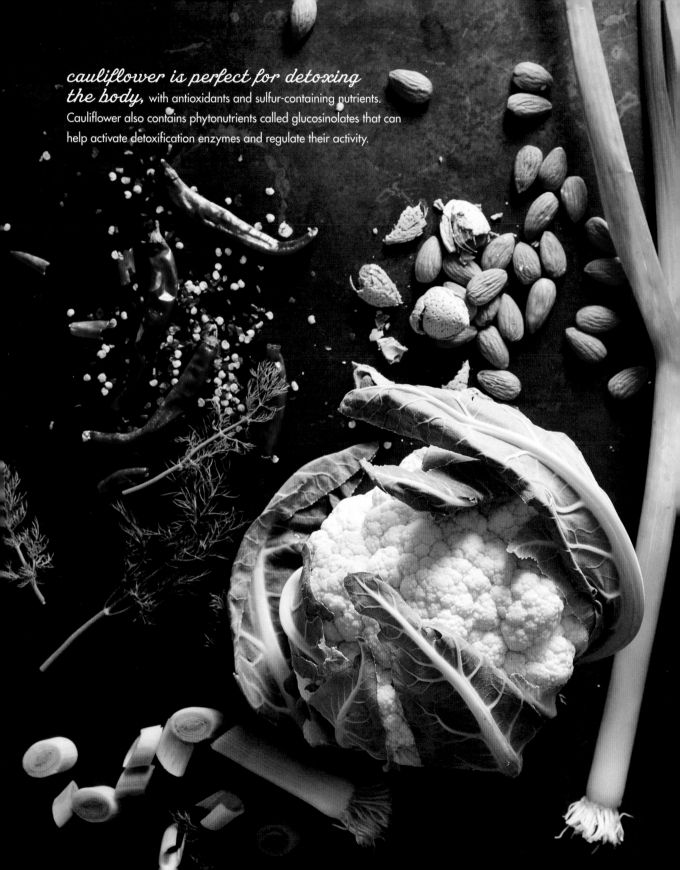

cauliflower is perfect for detoxing the body, with antioxidants and sulfur-containing nutrients. Cauliflower also contains phytonutrients called glucosinolates that can help activate detoxification enzymes and regulate their activity.

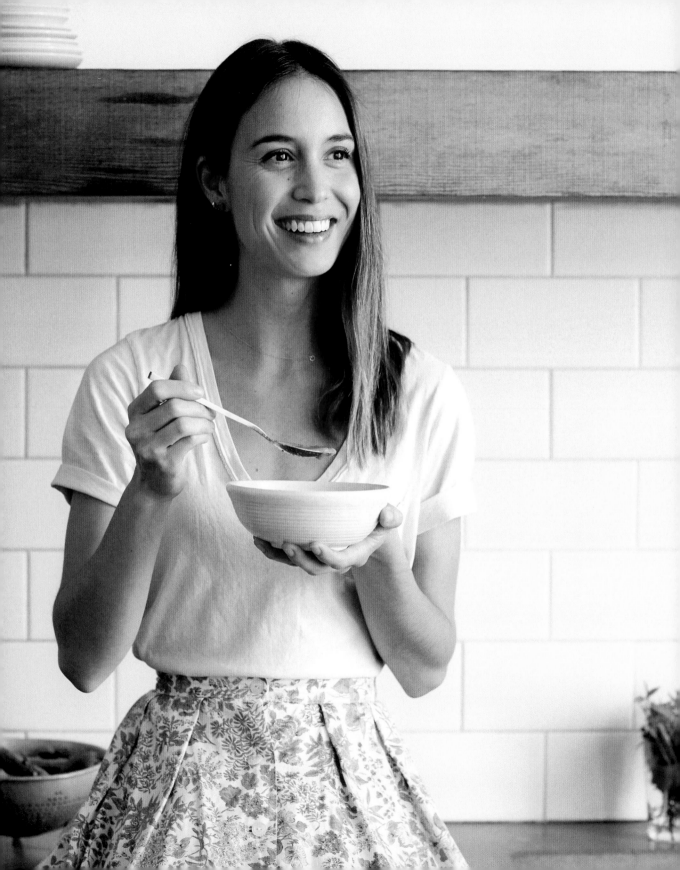

WHOLE CELERY PLANT

2 tablespoons olive oil

1 small yellow onion, diced

2 ribs celery, diced

1 large clove garlic, minced

2 sprigs fresh thyme, woody stems removed and leaves finely chopped

Pinch of ground black pepper

1 teaspoon sea salt

1½ pounds celeriac, peeled and diced

1 small russet potato, diced

1 cup leaves celery (whatever you can pull from the celery you have on hand)

1½ quarts water

1. In a medium pot over medium heat, warm the oil. Cook the onion, celery ribs, and garlic, stirring frequently, for 5 to 7 minutes, or until the vegetables are tender and translucent. Stir in the thyme, pepper, and salt and cook for 3 to 5 minutes, or until fragrant.

2. Add the celeriac, potato, and celery leaves and cook, stirring frequently, for 5 to 10 minutes, or until fragrant. (Leave a few celery leaves on the side as garnish.) Add the water, increase the heat to high, and bring to a boil. Reduce the heat to medium-high and simmer for 15 minutes.

3. Using an immersion blender or countertop blender, puree the soup until very smooth.

4. Pour into warm bowls and garnish with the extra celery leaves.

■ **WEIGHT LOSS**

Celery is one of those foods that people always think of when they think "diet" food. I've heard that it's a "negative-calorie" food, meaning it will take more calories to digest a piece of celery than the piece of celery contains. I've also heard that celery stimulates the same taste sensors that salt does, and that it can be a great substitute for a salt craving. I hardly think a celery stick will curb a craving for kettle-cooked potato chips, and a celery diet sounds like a boatload of no-fun. I was inspired more by my love for the unique flavor of celery. Celery's higher-pitched, somewhat-floral taste tickles my sinuses a bit, and much to my delight, the entire plant hums to the tune of this taste. The root is a softer, starchier celery flavor and texture; the stalks keep the tempo with that consistent beat of celery freshness; and the leaves are a final sweet chord that keeps your taste buds humming long after the last sip.

RAW CASHEW AND CUCUMBER

■ STRENGTHEN
■ MOM AND BABY
■ WEIGHT LOSS
■ DETOX

4 cups water, divided

1 cup quinoa

1 tablespoon olive oil

4 scallions, thinly sliced

1 large clove garlic, minced

¼ cup cashews, soaked in water overnight and drained (see "Why Soak Your Nuts and Seeds?" on page 74 for more information)

4 large cucumbers, peeled, seeded, and chopped

1 cup loosely packed and stripped fresh dill

1 cup loosely packed fresh mint leaves

2 tablespoons apple cider vinegar

Pinch of ground black pepper

½ teaspoon sea salt

1. In a small pot over high heat, bring 2 cups of the water to a boil. Reduce the heat to medium, add the quinoa, and simmer for 15 minutes. Drain and set aside.

2. In a small pan over medium heat, warm the oil. Cook the scallions and garlic, stirring, for 7 to 10 minutes, or until the mixture is very soft and sweet.

3. In a countertop blender, combine the scallion mixture, cashews, cucumbers, dill, mint, vinegar, pepper, and salt. Puree until very smooth, slowly adding the remaining 2 cups water as necessary to achieve a thin milkshake consistency. Cover and cool in the refrigerator for 1 hour.

4. Gently mound a quarter of the quinoa into the bottom of each bowl and ladle the soup on top.

I had a traditional cucumber soup in Istanbul called cacik that was so elegant I think of it every time the weather turns warm. It was creamy but refreshing, herbal, and a bit nutty from some barley. And my favorite part was that it came in a wide, shallow saucer dotted with round ice cubes. How exquisite! It felt like such a sophisticated way to enjoy soup—somehow more advanced than the warm stews and steamy broths we are accustomed to at home. This version contains no dairy (of course) but the flavor is just as creamy as the cacik in Turkey because of the cashew cream.

the cucumber soup i had in turkey had barley in it, but I like making my soups gluten-free for all my friends with celiac disease and gluten intolerance—and there are more with these issues every day it seems! Quinoa—a seed that adds texture, protein, and essential minerals—is widely available now. See, everyone's happy.

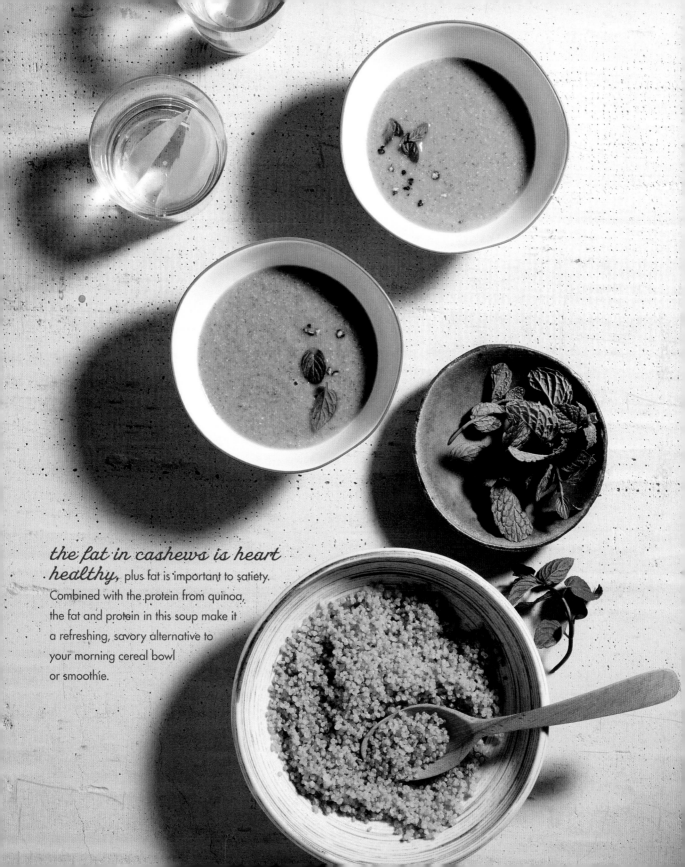

the fat in cashews is heart healthy, plus fat is important to satiety. Combined with the protein from quinoa, the fat and protein in this soup make it a refreshing, savory alternative to your morning cereal bowl or smoothie.

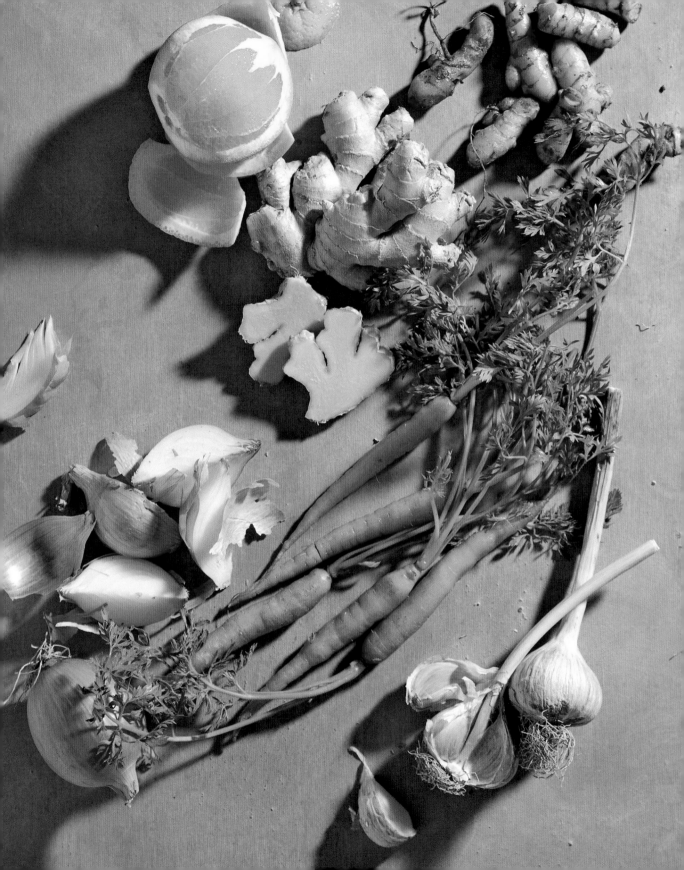

CARROT *and* TURMERIC

1 tablespoon olive oil

1 yellow onion, diced

1 clove garlic, minced

1 large bunch carrots, cut into 2" chunks (about 2 pounds)

1 teaspoon chopped fresh rosemary

1 tablespoon freshly grated turmeric or 1 teaspoon ground

1 tablespoon grated fresh ginger or 1 teaspoon ground

1 quart water plus 2 cups as needed

Grated peel and juice of 2 oranges

Pinch of ground red pepper

Pinch of ground black pepper

Pinch of sea salt

1. In a large pot over medium heat, warm the oil. Cook the onion and garlic, stirring, for 5 minutes, or until the mixture is soft and translucent. Add the carrots, rosemary, turmeric, and ginger and stir to combine.

2. Reduce the heat to medium-low and add the 1 quart water, orange peel, and orange juice. Cover and simmer for about 25 minutes. Add the red pepper, black pepper, and salt.

3. Using an immersion blender or countertop blender, puree the soup until very smooth, adding the remaining 2 cups water as needed to reach this consistency.

4. Portion into 4 separate containers and leave uncovered in the refrigerator to chill for 2 hours before enjoying.

■ DETOX
■ ENERGIZE
■ HEAL
■ WEIGHT LOSS

This bright orange soup is brimming with beta-carotene, which intensifies as you cook it. Fresh turmeric enhances the health quotient of this soup: Its anti-inflammatory properties are activated with ground black pepper and the heat from your stove. This is one of our classic flavors at Splendid Spoon, and it is a fan favorite to start the morning. The ginger is like a boisterous clap awakening you to the day ahead.

SPRING PEA WITH CASHEW CREAM

Peas are in the legume family, and they are a wonderful source of both protein and fiber. This soup has the magical effect of tasting light while also keeping you full for hours. It's a glorious green color that will make your lips smack for a longer season of spring.

1 tablespoon olive oil

4 scallions, roughly chopped

1 clove garlic, chopped

1½ pounds shelled English peas or frozen green peas, about 5 cups (see note)

2 cups water plus 2 cups as needed

Pinch of ground black pepper

Pinch of sea salt

Peel of ½ lemon, grated (about 1 teaspoon)

Juice of ½ lemon

1 tablespoon chopped fresh mint

1 quart ice

¼ cup cashews, soaked in water overnight and drained (see "Why Soak Your Nuts and Seeds?" on page 74 for more information)

1. In a large pot over medium heat, warm the oil. Cook the scallions and garlic for 3 minutes, or until the mixture is soft and translucent.

2. Stir in the peas, 2 cups of the water, pepper, and salt, cover, and cook for about 8 minutes. (If using frozen peas, cook for about 5 minutes.)

3. Remove the pot from the stove. Add the lemon peel, lemon juice, mint, and ice. Using an immersion blender or countertop blender, puree for 3 to 4 minutes, or until very smooth and cool, adding the remaining water as needed to reach this consistency.

4. In a countertop blender or food processor, combine the cashews with ¼ cup of the remaining water. Blend until smooth.

5. Serve immediately in a chilled bowl with a dollop of the cashew cream.

Note: English peas are the roly-poly peas that you pop out of their tougher outer shells. Many stores will also sell the peas preshelled. I list the final shelled weight. Peas with an edible outer shell, like sugar snap peas and snow peas, don't work as well in this recipe.

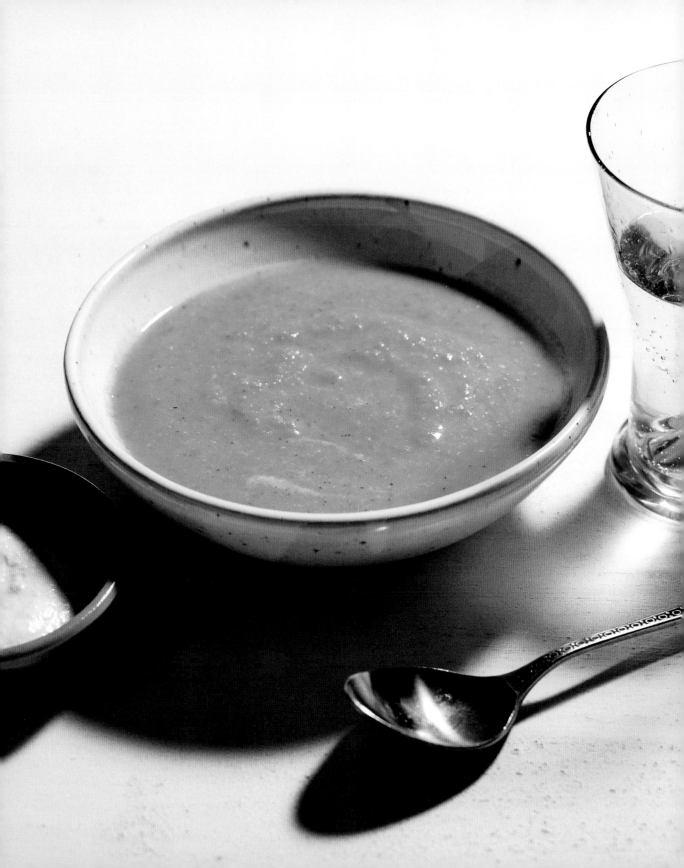

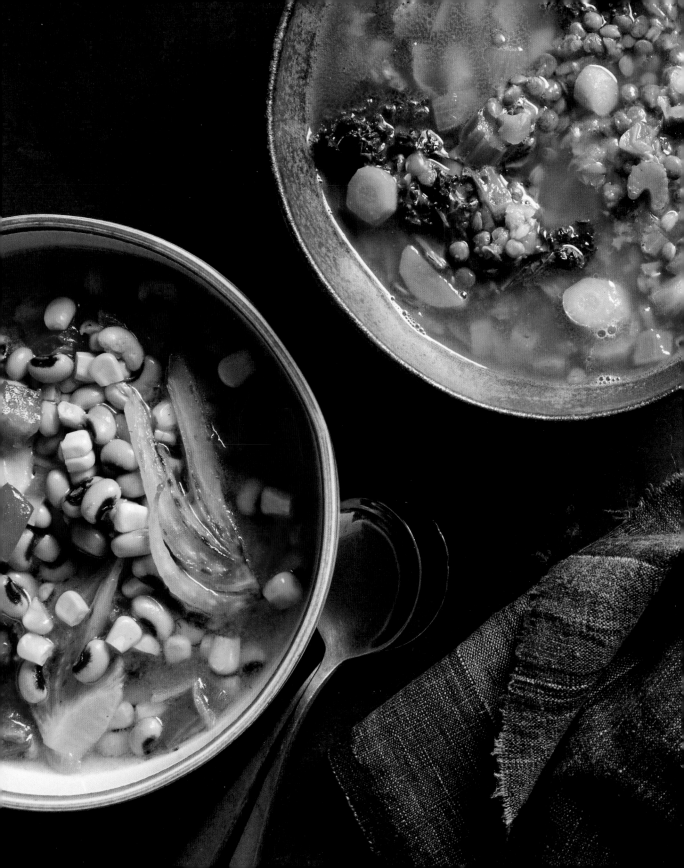

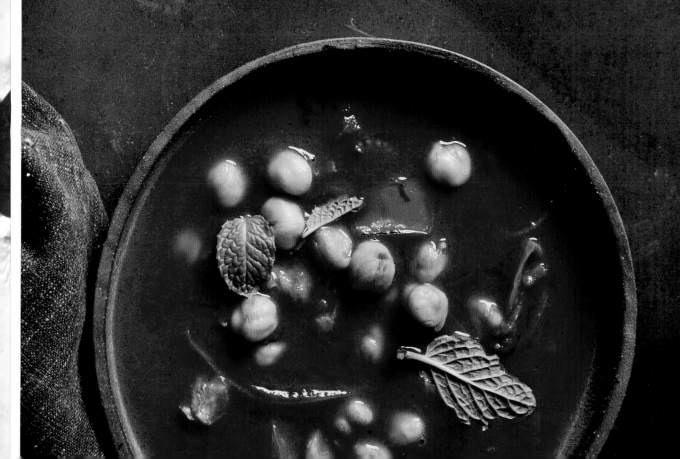

chapter 6

BEANS
AND LENTILS

CHICKPEA STEW

■ WEIGHT LOSS
■ STRENGTHEN
■ MOM AND BABY

2 tablespoons olive oil

4 scallions, thinly sliced

1 rib celery, diced

1 large clove garlic, chopped

¾ teaspoon ground cumin

½ teaspoon ground black pepper

2 large tomatoes, chopped, or ½ can (7 ounces) diced tomatoes

½ pound dried chickpeas, soaked overnight and drained, or 2 cans (15 ounces each) low-sodium chickpeas

1½ quarts water (reduce to 1 quart if using canned beans)

Peel of 2 limes, grated (about 4 teaspoons)

Juice of 2 limes

1½ teaspoons sea salt (omit if using canned beans)

1 cup loosely packed fresh cilantro

A fiber and protein power-house, this hearty stew will strengthen and satisfy. Smooth and buttery with a hint of sweetness, chickpeas (or garbanzo beans) provide a rich flavor complemented by brightly acidic tomatoes, earthy cumin, and the herbal freshness of cilantro.

1. In a medium pot over medium heat, warm the oil. Cook the scallions, celery, and garlic, stirring, for 3 minutes, or until the mixture is soft. Stir in the cumin and pepper and cook for 5 minutes, or until fragrant.

2. Add the tomatoes and chickpeas and cook, stirring, for 5 minutes, or until the tomatoes begin to reduce. Increase the heat to high, add the water, and bring to a boil. Partially cover the mixture, allowing some steam to escape, reduce the heat to low, and simmer for 1 hour and 30 minutes, or until the chickpeas are very tender. If using canned beans, cook, uncovered, for 30 minutes, or until the water is reduced and the soup has thickened.

3. Using an immersion blender, pulse until some of the starch thickens the broth but there are still whole chickpeas. Or puree a quarter of the mixture in a countertop blender and then add back to the pot.

4. Stir in the lime peel, lime juice, salt, and cilantro and serve warm or chilled.

you've probably heard of the soapy cilantro phenomenon, where our favorite bright herb tastes like a bar of soap to some people. Why does this happen? Some of us have olfactory-receptor genes that can distinguish the flavor of aldehyde chemicals—strangely found in both cilantro and soap. If this is you, don't flip the page just yet. You can always substitute parsley instead to eliminate any soapy flavors!

MUNG *and* QUINOA CONGEE

1 cup diced eggplant (about ½ eggplant)

2 teaspoons sea salt, divided for eggplant and seasoning (omit the 1 teaspoon for seasoning if using canned beans)

1 tablespoon sesame oil

4 cloves garlic, sliced

1 small onion, diced

1 rib celery, diced

½ teaspoon ground black pepper

2½ quarts water (reduce to 1 quart if using canned beans)

1 cup mung beans, rinsed and drained (pick out small stones), or ½ can (7.5 ounces) pigeon beans, rinsed and drained

½ cup quinoa, rinsed and drained

2 cups spinach, torn into bite-size pieces

1. Place the eggplant in a strainer over a bowl. Toss with 1 teaspoon of the salt. Let sit while you prepare the other vegetables and cook the garlic.

2. Meanwhile, in a medium pot over medium heat, warm the oil. Cook the garlic for 2 to 3 minutes, or until fragrant. Turn off the heat.

3. Rinse the salted eggplant under running water and squeeze the cubes gently with your hands to remove as much moisture as possible.

4. In the same pot over medium heat, add the onion, celery, eggplant, and pepper and cook, stirring frequently, for 10 minutes, or until the vegetables are tender.

5. Stir in the water, beans, and quinoa. Increase the heat to high and bring to a boil. Reduce the heat to low, cover, and simmer for 45 minutes, or until the beans are very tender or split open. If using canned beans, simmer for 20 minutes.

6. Stir in the spinach and the remaining 1 teaspoon of salt, cover, and cook for 5 minutes, or until the spinach is wilted.

mung beans are a staple in Ayurvedic practice—an ancient Indian wellness philosophy that embraces the mind-body connection and encourages a simple whole-food diet with lots of cooked vegetables. Mung beans are high in soluble and insoluble fiber, which helps keep your digestive tract and blood vessels clear.

■ ENERGIZE
■ STRENGTHEN
■ MOM AND BABY

The first time I had congee was on a 24-hour flight to the Philippines. Yes, airplane congee. Even in the reheated dish with the foil cover and plastic spoon, this meal was flavorful, satisfying, and fragrant. Congee first appeared around 1000 BC, during the Zhou Dynasty in China, and its powers to comfort and fortify continue today. Traditionally, it gets a porridge texture from long-cooked white rice, but I achieve a similar texture with nutrient-dense mung beans and quinoa. I love this soup, savory and steeped in rich flavor, for its delicate blend of softly sweet mung beans and nutty quinoa. Spinach satisfies your need for something green with its serious and dense cooked flavor.

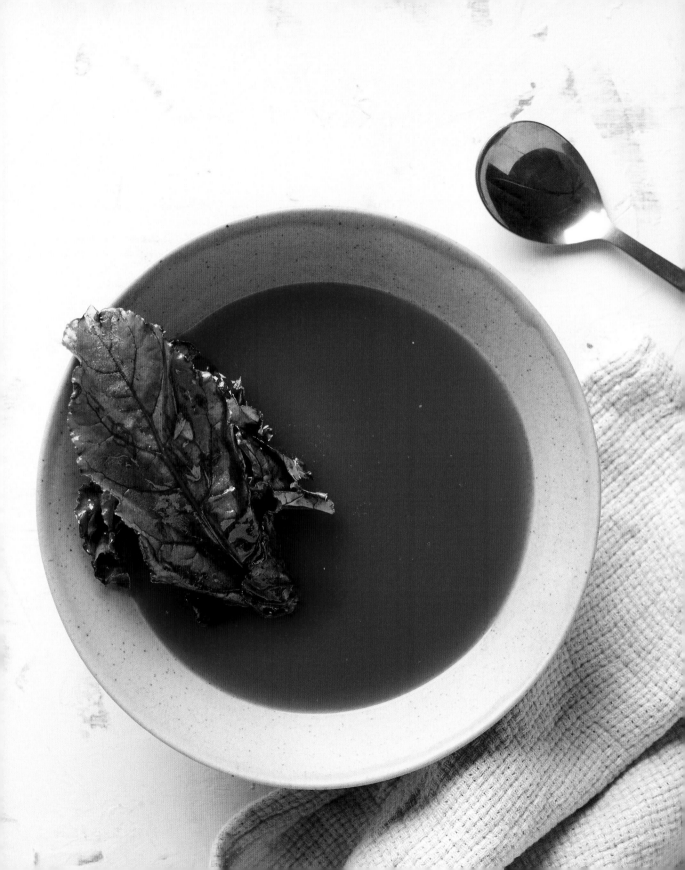

WHITE BEAN PUREE *with* BEETS *and* BEET GREENS

■ MOM AND BABY
■ STRENGTHEN
■ DETOX

This luscious puree has a nutty earthiness from the white beans, and it includes deep ruby-red beets and their bold, slightly bitter greens, whose flavor is reminiscent of kale. Enjoy this soup for its high concentration of folate and the phytochemical betaine, which improves vascular health. Since Roman times, beetroot juice has been considered an aphrodisiac. Consider any amorous feelings a happy side effect!

1	tablespoon olive oil
1	small onion, sliced
1	large clove garlic, minced
2	beets with greens, greens removed and sliced and beets diced (don't worry about removing the peel)
1	carrot, diced
½	pound dried white beans (navy or cannellini), soaked overnight and drained, or ½ can (7.5 ounces) low-sodium navy beans, rinsed and drained
1½	quarts water (reduce to 1 quart if using canned beans)
1	teaspoon grated orange peel
	Pinch of sea salt (omit if using canned beans)
	Pinch of ground black pepper

1. In a medium pot over medium heat, warm the oil. Cook the onion and garlic, stirring frequently, for 5 to 7 minutes, or until the mixture is tender and translucent.

2. Stir in the beet greens and cook, tossing frequently, for 7 minutes, or until wilted. Remove the greens and set aside. (Some of the onion and garlic will come with the greens, and that's perfectly fine!)

3. Add the carrot and beets to the pot and cook, stirring, for 5 minutes, or until fragrant. Add the beans and water and bring to a boil. Cover and simmer for 2 hours (45 minutes if using canned beans), or until the beans and beets are very tender. (Or use a slow cooker overnight on low.)

4. Take the pot off the heat and add the orange peel, salt, and pepper. Using an immersion blender or countertop blender, puree the soup until very smooth. (Don't worry about the beet skin; peeling it off will burn your fingers at this point, and root vegetables hold on to lots of nutrients just below the skin.)

5. Ladle the soup into a warm bowl and top with some of the reserved greens. Store any leftover soup and greens separately.

beet greens are a rich source of iron. As a member of the dark leafy green vegetables, these greens stand apart from the crowd as an incredible source of minerals, including high levels of both calcium and magnesium. It's a rarity to find such large amounts of both. Just 1 serving of beet greens provides 25 percent of the RDI (Reference Daily Intake) of magnesium.

BELL PEPPER BISQUE

2 tablespoons olive oil

1 small onion, sliced

1 large clove garlic, chopped

2 large tomatoes, chopped, or ½ can (7 ounces) diced tomatoes

½ pound dried white beans (navy or cannellini), soaked overnight and drained, or 2 cans (15 ounces each) low-sodium white beans, rinsed and drained

1½ quarts water (reduce to 1 quart if using canned beans)

½ cup roasted red peppers, chopped (see "Roast Your Own Peppers" to roast yourself or use high-quality jarred peppers like Divina, which are widely available)

2 teaspoons sea salt (omit if using canned beans)

½ cup loosely packed fresh basil, torn

Sweetly roasted red bell peppers are the crown jewels of this beautiful bisque, with green basil, fresh tomatoes, and smooth white beans blended together to create a soup that's both creamy and savory.

1. In a medium pot over medium heat, warm the oil. Cook the onion and garlic, stirring frequently, for 4 minutes, or until the mixture is soft and translucent.

2. Stir in the tomatoes, beans, and water and bring to a boil. Reduce the heat to medium-low, cover, and simmer for 2 hours, or until the beans are very tender. If using canned beans, cook for about 20 minutes, or until heated through.

3. In a countertop blender, combine the soup, peppers, salt, and basil. Puree until very smooth. Do this in batches, if necessary, and remember to vent the lid slightly to allow steam to escape. Enjoy warm or chilled.

ROAST YOUR OWN PEPPERS

To roast your own bell peppers, simply turn on the flame of your gas stove or turn on the broiler of a gas or electric stove. Here's your opportunity to really play with fire and char your veggies (don't worry, you won't be ingesting any of that char, though). Place the bell pepper directly on the burner of your stove or directly under the heat source of your broiler. You want the skin of the pepper to blister and blacken. Turn the pepper until it is blackened all the way around. This will take about 15 minutes of turning. Allow the pepper to cool before handling, and then peel and discard the burnt skin. It can be helpful to rub the skin with a dish towel if it isn't peeling easily. The more charred the skin, the easier to peel. Remove and discard the seeds before cooking with your roasted pepper. A roasted pepper has a sweeter, more concentrated flavor than a tangy raw pepper.

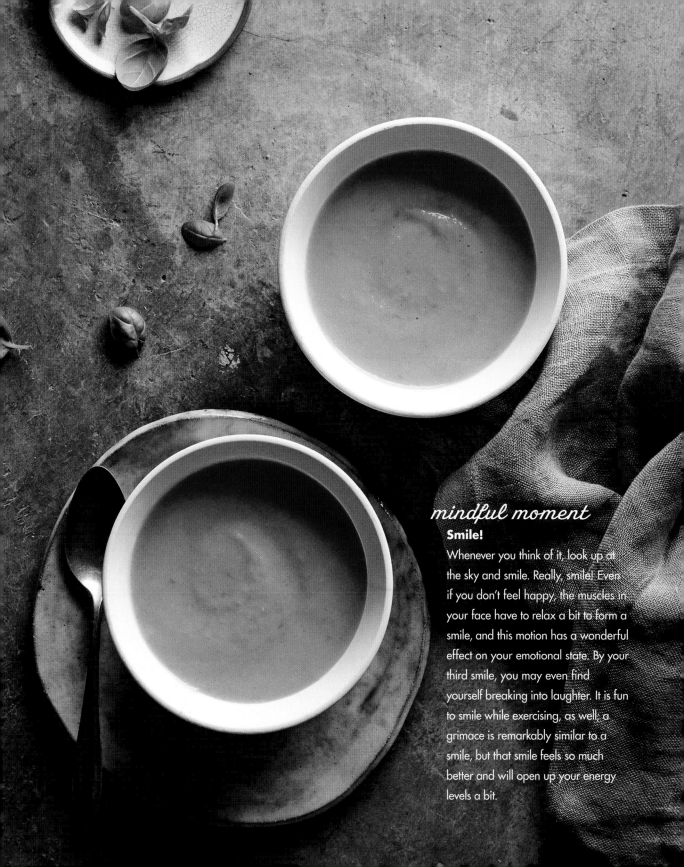

mindful moment
Smile!

Whenever you think of it, look up at the sky and smile. Really, smile! Even if you don't feel happy, the muscles in your face have to relax a bit to form a smile, and this motion has a wonderful effect on your emotional state. By your third smile, you may even find yourself breaking into laughter. It is fun to smile while exercising, as well; a grimace is remarkably similar to a smile, but that smile feels so much better and will open up your energy levels a bit.

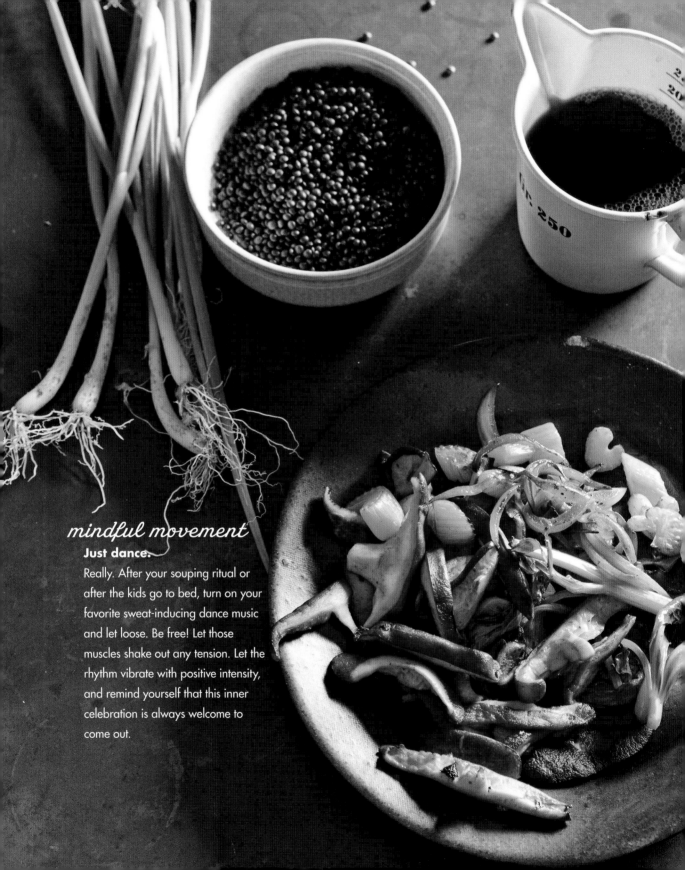

mindful movement

Just dance.

Really. After your souping ritual or after the kids go to bed, turn on your favorite sweat-inducing dance music and let loose. Be free! Let those muscles shake out any tension. Let the rhythm vibrate with positive intensity, and remind yourself that this inner celebration is always welcome to come out.

BLACK LENTILS WITH COFFEE *and* SHIITAKES

Hear me out if you're suspicious of this savory java soup. The bitter acidity of coffee provides a sharp contrasting flavor to the smooth lentils and rich, meaty shiitakes.

1 small onion, diced

1 rib celery, diced

2 cups thinly sliced shiitake caps (about 3.5 ounces)

2 tablespoons coconut oil, melted

1½ quarts water

1 cup brewed black coffee

1 pound dried black or beluga lentils, rinsed and drained (pick out small stones)

½ teaspoon ground black pepper

1 scallion, sliced

1. Preheat the oven to 425°F.

2. On a baking sheet, toss the onion, celery, and shiitake caps with the oil and spread into a single layer. Roast for 25 minutes, stirring halfway through, or until soft and browned.

3. Meanwhile, in a medium pot over high heat, bring the water and coffee to a boil. Stir in the lentils and pepper. Reduce the heat to low, cover, and simmer for 25 minutes, or until the lentils are soft but still firm.

4. Stir in the mushroom mixture and cook, covered, for 10 minutes. Garnish with the scallion slices and serve hot or chilled.

PLANT-BASED BULLETPROOF COFFEE
Speaking of coffee, here's a recipe for my favorite way to enjoy this very popular beverage. In a countertop blender, combine 1 cup hot coffee with ¾ teaspoon coconut oil, ½ teaspoon ground cinnamon, and 1 tablespoon soaked almonds. Blend until very smooth and frothy. Yum!

SESAME BLACK BEAN CHILI

There are few things more satisfying on a cold winter night than curling up with a steaming bowl of chili. This recipe combines protein-rich black beans, a medley of spices and seeds, and the subtle heat of jalapeño peppers to create a classic, hearty chili with a nutty twist of sesame.

1 tablespoon olive oil

1 tablespoon sesame oil

1 small onion, sliced

2 large cloves garlic, chopped

1 tablespoon tomato paste

1 jalapeño pepper, seeded and finely chopped (use gloves if your skin is sensitive to hot peppers)

1 teaspoon ground cumin

1 teaspoon sweet paprika

¼ teaspoon ground black pepper

4 large tomatoes, chopped, or 1 can (14 ounces) diced tomatoes

½ pound black beans, soaked overnight and drained, or 2 cans (15 ounces each) low-sodium black beans, rinsed and drained

2 quarts water (reduce to 1 quart if using canned beans)

2 teaspoons sea salt (omit if using canned beans)

½ cup chopped fresh cilantro

¼ cup toasted sesame seeds

Lime wedges (optional)

1. In a medium pot over medium heat, warm the oils. Cook the onion, garlic, tomato paste, jalapeño pepper, cumin, paprika, and black pepper, stirring frequently, for 5 minutes, or until the onion and garlic are tender and translucent.

2. Stir in the tomatoes and cook 5 to 7 minutes, or until the tomatoes are darker in color and some of the tomato juice has reduced.

3. Stir in the beans and water. Increase the heat to high and bring to a boil. Reduce the heat to low, cover, and simmer for 2 hours, or until the beans are very tender. If using canned beans, cook, uncovered, for 45 minutes, or until the water is reduced and the soup has thickened. Stir in the salt.

4. Garnish with the cilantro, sesame seeds, and lime wedges (if using).

the sesame seed's history is as rich as its distinctive flavor. The oldest domesticated oil seed crop, dating back 5,000 years, sesame seeds originated in sub-Saharan Africa and India.

RED CHILI

3 tablespoons olive oil

1 small onion, sliced

2 large cloves garlic, minced

1 red bell pepper, diced (about 1 cup)

2 chipotle peppers, seeded and chopped, or canned in adobe sauce, chopped

1 teaspoon ground Aleppo pepper or ½ teaspoon ground red pepper

½ pound dried kidney beans, soaked overnight and drained, or 2 cans (15 ounces each) low-sodium kidney beans, rinsed and drained

2 large tomatoes, chopped, or ½ can (7 ounces) diced tomatoes

2 quarts water (reduce to 1 quart if using canned beans)

1 teaspoon sea salt (omit if using canned beans)

¼ cup chopped fresh mint

¼ cup toasted almond slivers

The iconic kidney bean is named for its shape. It's a fiber-rich flavor sponge that absorbs the diverse flavors of its surroundings. In this soup, it imparts the rich flavors of simmered Aleppo and chipotle peppers, luscious olive oil, garlic, and freshly chopped mint into every spoonful.

1. In a medium pot over medium heat, warm the oil. Cook the onion, garlic, bell pepper, chipotle peppers, and Aleppo or red pepper, stirring frequently, for 5 minutes, or until the onion and garlic are tender and translucent.

2. Stir in the beans, tomatoes, and water. Increase the heat to high and bring to a boil. Reduce the heat to low, cover, and simmer for 2 hours, or until the beans are very tender. If using canned beans, cook, uncovered, for 45 minutes, or until the water is reduced and the soup has thickened. Stir in the salt.

3. Garnish with the mint and toasted almonds.

the aleppo pepper is sometimes called a halaby pepper, but the distinctive burgundy hue is constant, regardless of what you call it. High in antioxidants and vitamin A (those rich red hues mean lots of carotenoids!), this pepper can aid in cardiovascular health. It has also been used as an expectorant due to the pepper's mucus-thinning properties, which just means if you have some congestion and want to get the gunk out of your respiratory system, the Aleppo pepper might help your coughs be more, ahem, productive.

GREEN CHILI

■ ENERGIZE
■ WEIGHT LOSS
■ STRENGTHEN
■ DETOX
■ MOM AND BABY

3 tablespoons olive oil, divided

1 small onion, sliced

2 large cloves garlic, minced, divided

½ pound dried white beans (navy or cannellini), soaked overnight and drained, or 2 cans (15 ounces each) low-sodium white beans, rinsed and drained

2 quarts water (reduce to 1 quart if using canned beans)

1 jalapeño pepper, seeded and chopped (use gloves if your skin is sensitive to hot peppers)

2 teaspoons sea salt (omit if using canned beans)

1 teaspoon white wine vinegar

¼ cup chopped fresh dill

¼ cup chopped fresh flat-leaf parsley

¼ cup chopped fresh cilantro

¼ cup chopped fresh basil

You've heard of white, red, and black chili, but this green goddess is sure to raise the bar for chilis of all hues. Its bright medley of herbs (dill, parsley, cilantro, and basil!) gives a fresh, innovative flavor to an otherwise classic, hearty bean soup.

1. In a medium pot over medium heat, warm 1 tablespoon of the oil. Cook the onion and half of the garlic, stirring frequently, for 5 minutes, or until the mixture is tender and translucent.

2. Stir in the beans and water. Increase the heat to high and bring to a boil. Reduce the heat to low, cover, and simmer for 2 hours, or until the beans are very tender. If using canned beans, cook, uncovered, for 30 minutes, or until the water is reduced and the soup has thickened.

3. Meanwhile, in a food processor, puree the pepper, salt, vinegar, dill, parsley, cilantro, basil, the remaining garlic, and the remaining 2 tablespoons oil.

4. Stir the herb mixture into the cooked beans just before serving.

cool, green, and delicate, dill brings more to a dish than just its signature flavor and pretty fronds. Dill oil prevents bacterial growth, making it the cleanest herb around. Dill also combats free radicals through the healing components of monoterpenes (which counteract oxidation of cells) and flavonoids (plant metabolites that have antioxidant effects).

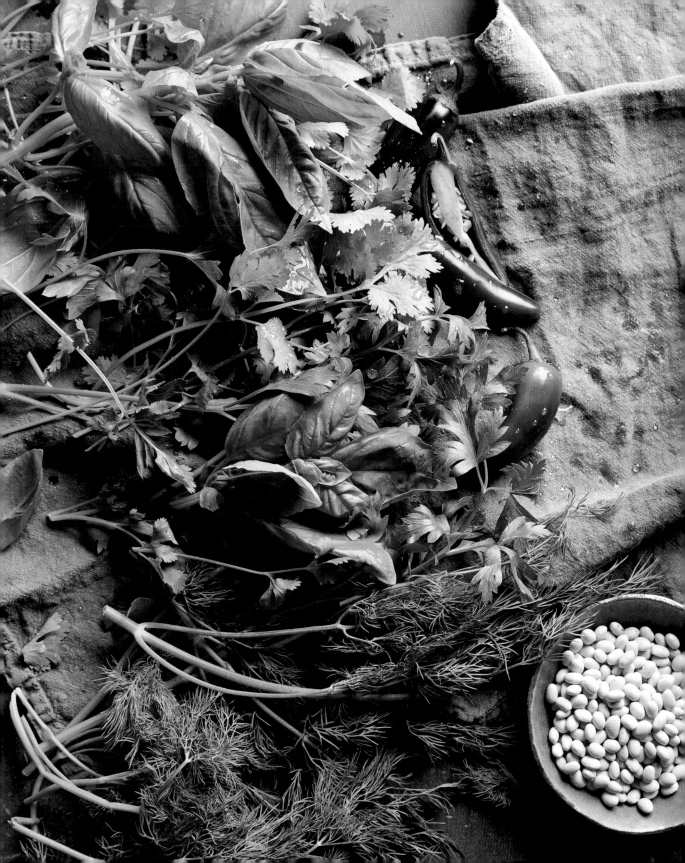

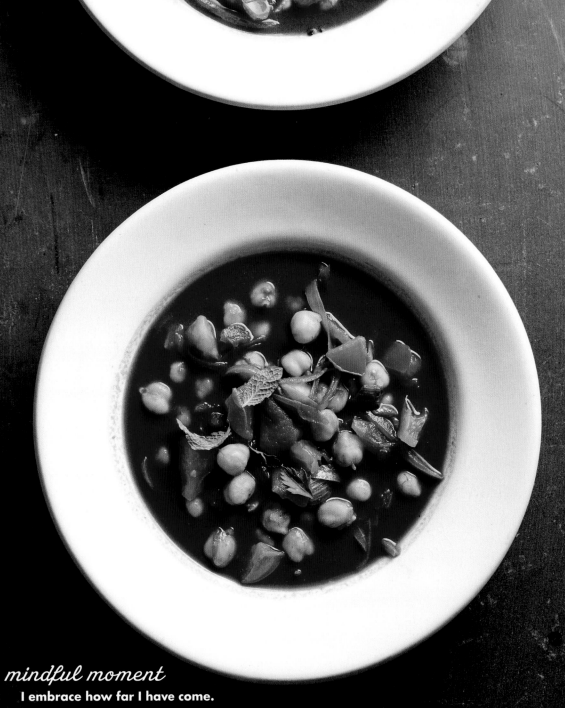

mindful moment

I embrace how far I have come.

Whether you have been souping for a day, a week, a month, or a year, the passage of time is happening constantly, and it is important to acknowledge it. Be joyful that you are moving always and that each time you choose to sit down for your souping ritual, you are moving in a direction of your own positive design.

PLANT-BASED TAGINE

2 tablespoons olive oil

1 small onion, chopped

1 rib celery, chopped

1 large clove garlic, minced

2 large tomatoes, chopped, or ½ can (7 ounces) diced tomatoes, including the juice

1 cup chopped fresh apricots or ½ cup dried, soaked in 1 cup hot water and drained and chopped, divided

1 tablespoon tomato paste

½ teaspoon ground cumin

½ teaspoon ground black pepper

1 tablespoon 100% cocoa powder

½ pound dried chickpeas, soaked overnight and drained, or 2 cans (15 ounces each) low-sodium chickpeas, rinsed and drained

2 quarts plus 1 cup water (reduce to 1 quart if using canned beans)

½ cup almonds, soaked overnight and drained (see "Why Soak Your Nuts and Seeds?" on page 74 for more information)

1½ teaspoons sea salt (omit if using canned beans)

½ cup loosely packed fresh flat-leaf parsley

¼ cup loosely packed fresh mint

1. In a medium pot over medium heat, warm the oil. Cook the onion and celery for 5 to 7 minutes, or until the mixture is tender and translucent. Stir in the garlic and cook for 1 minute, or until fragrant.

2. Stir in the tomatoes, half of the apricots, the tomato paste, cumin, pepper, cocoa powder, chickpeas, and 2 quarts of the water. Increase the heat to high and bring to a boil. Reduce the heat to low, cover (leaving a vent for air to escape), and simmer for 1 hour, or until the chickpeas are very tender. If using canned beans, cook, uncovered, for 30 minutes, or until the water is reduced and the soup has thickened.

3. Meanwhile, using an immersion blender or countertop blender, puree the almonds with the remaining 1 cup water.

4. Stir the salt, parsley, mint, and almond "cream" into the pot.

5. Serve warm or chilled garnished with the remaining apricots.

■ ENERGIZE
■ HEAL
■ WEIGHT LOSS
■ STRENGTHEN
■ DETOX
■ MOM AND BABY

This rich stew is the "plantified" version of the classic Moroccan dish often featuring lamb, beef, chicken, or fish as well as an assortment of vegetables and spices. Here, the vegetables take center stage with all of their rich, wonderful flavors. Fresh herbs and a surprising dash of cocoa powder complete this delicious mosaic of flavor.

Tagine has as much to do with the vessel it is cooked in as it does with the stew ingredients. A traditional tagine is cooked in a conical clay pot with a wide shallow bowl and cone-shaped lid—kind of the Dutch oven of Northern Africa.

mindful mantra

Growth is synonymous with change.

I trust my ability to change. Change is not easy.

Regardless of the change—trying to get up earlier for a workout, quitting a longstanding habit, or even remembering a new school or work schedule—our bodies often resist the change and try to stay on their original paths. Reciting this mantra will deepen your appreciation for your ability to change. Growth only happens with change and change is hard, but you can do it, and it starts with trusting yourself. Repeat this mantra every time you prepare your soup, eat your soup, share your soup, and reach for soup instead of ordering takeout or grabbing a sugary granola bar.

CHILLED CHICKPEA-AVOCADO TAHINI PUREE

Sure you've had avocado on toast, in smoothies, and scooped up in guacamole, but have you tried it in *soup*? This versatile fruit steals the show in an ultra-creamy puree of mild, nutty chickpeas and tahini blended seamlessly with ripe avocado—one of the best plant fats around. Add in freshly chopped chives for a bright crispness and a zesty splash of lemon or lime juice to balance the creaminess with a bite of citric acid.

½ pound dried chickpeas, soaked overnight and drained, or 1 can (15 ounces) low-sodium chickpeas, rinsed and drained

1½ quarts water plus more as needed (reduce to 1 quart if using canned beans)

1 cup ice

2 tablespoons tahini

1 tablespoon chopped fresh chives

3 very ripe avocados, halved and flesh scooped out

Peel of 1 lemon, grated (about 2 teaspoons)

Juice of 1 lemon

Peel of 1 lime, grated (about 2 teaspoons)

Juice of 1 lime

1½ teaspoons sea salt (omit if using canned beans)

1. In a medium pot over medium-high heat, simmer the chickpeas and water for 25 minutes, or until the chickpeas are very tender. Drain the liquid. (Skip this step if using canned chickpeas.)

2. In a countertop blender, add the chickpeas, ice, tahini, chives, avocados, lemon peel, lemon juice, lime peel, lime juice, and salt. Blend until a smoothielike consistency, adding more water as needed.

tahini is a condiment made of toasted sesame seeds that are hulled and ground into an oily paste. (The Arabic word *tahini* means "to grind.") Tahini has more protein than milk and many nuts. It's also a great source of vitamin E, which guards against heart disease and stroke, as well as a nondairy source for calcium.

CARROT COCONUT CURRY

2 tablespoons coconut oil

1 small onion, diced

1 rib celery, diced

4 cups chopped carrots

1 clove garlic, minced

2 tablespoons Madras curry powder

½ pound dried black lentils, rinsed and drained (pick out small stones)

2 quarts water

1 can (15 ounces) coconut milk

1½ teaspoons sea salt

½ cup chopped fresh cilantro

Pinch of red-pepper flakes

Peel of 1 orange, grated (optional)

This is the curry of your coconut dreams, with luscious coconut oil and coconut milk to impart a sweet nuttiness to this vegetable-rich curry. Carrots and Madras curry add a bright golden-orange color that contrasts with hearty black lentils and bold red-pepper flakes.

1. In a medium pot over medium heat, warm the oil. Cook the onion, celery, and carrots, stirring frequently, for 10 minutes, or until the mixture is tender. Stir in the garlic and curry and cook for 1 minute, or until fragrant.

2. Stir in the lentils, water, coconut milk, and salt and cook for 25 minutes, or until the lentils are tender but still al dente.

3. Enjoy warm or chilled. Garnish with the cilantro, red-pepper flakes, and orange peel (if using).

coconut oil is all the rage these days, from oil pulling for dental health to my Plant-Based Bulletproof Coffee for a velvety jolt of caffeine (a favorite at our office, recipe on page 97). But its origins date well back to 4,000 years ago. The coconut has been a staple in tropical cultures for its milk, flesh, water, and oil. Because of its high level of plant-based saturated fat (the good kind!), coconut oil acts as a buttery solid at room temperature and a rich oil when heated; it's great for frying and popping popcorn as it can withstand high levels of heat without forming free radicals, like many polyunsaturated oils.

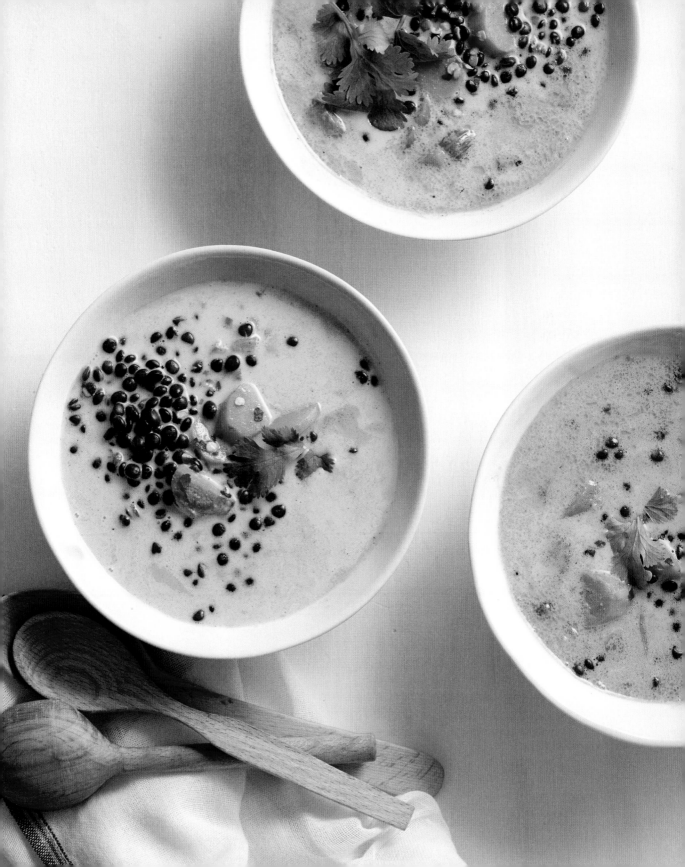

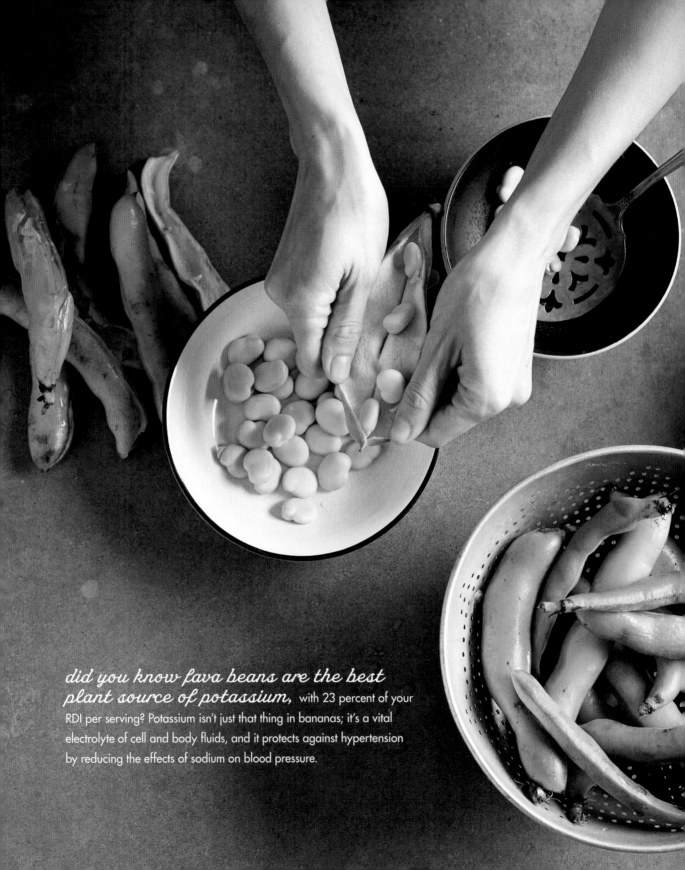

did you know fava beans are the best plant source of potassium, with 23 percent of your RDI per serving? Potassium isn't just that thing in bananas; it's a vital electrolyte of cell and body fluids, and it protects against hypertension by reducing the effects of sodium on blood pressure.

SPRING FAVAS *with* ASPARAGUS, LEMON, *and* DILL

Like walking through a springtime garden, this soup is a delicate bouquet of zesty citrus, tangy dill, fresh mint, and crunchy green asparagus. Fava beans add nourishing protein and heartiness to this beautifully blooming soup.

2 tablespoons olive oil

3 stalks green garlic, chopped, or 1 bunch scallions, sliced, or 1 clove garlic, minced

1 cup fresh fava beans (remove the beans from the pod and then remove the bright green beans from their opaque outer casings) or frozen lima beans

1½ quarts water

2 teaspoons sea salt

1 bunch asparagus, woody ends removed and tender parts shaved into ribbons

Juice of 1 lemon

¼ cup chopped fresh dill

1 tablespoon chopped fresh mint

1. In a medium pot over medium-high heat, warm the oil. Cook the green garlic or scallions or garlic for 6 minutes, or until tender.

2. Add the fava beans or lima beans, water, and salt and simmer for 10 minutes, or until the beans are tender. Add the asparagus and cook for 3 to 4 minutes, or until the asparagus is cooked through.

3. Turn off the heat and stir in the lemon juice, dill, and mint. Serve warm with a drizzle of olive oil.

green garlic is simply immature garlic and looks like a slightly overgrown scallion or green onion. Look for green garlic plants with fresh green tops (no dried ends or soggy leaves). To use, trim off the root ends and any tough parts of the green leaves. Chop or slice the white and light green parts and the first few inches of the dark green leaves (as long as they are tender). Use as you would scallions or regular garlic, noting that it is stronger than the former but milder than the latter.

BLACK-EYED PEA SUCCOTASH

■ ENERGIZE
■ STRENGTHEN

This popular Southern dish combines hearty black-eyed peas, sweet yellow corn, acidic tomatoes, bright fennel, and tangy dill to produce a bounty of flavor.

- 1   tablespoon olive oil
- 1   small onion, diced
- ½   bulb fennel, diced
- 1   large clove garlic, minced
- ½   pound dried black-eyed peas, soaked overnight and drained, or 1 can (15 ounces) black-eyed peas, rinsed and drained
- 1½ quarts water (reduce to 1 quart if using canned beans)
- ½   cup corn (about 1 cob's worth of kernels)
- 2   large tomatoes, diced, or ½ can (7 ounces) diced tomatoes
- ½   teaspoon ground black pepper
- 1   teaspoon sea salt (omit if using canned beans)
- ½   cup chopped fresh dill

1. In a medium pot over medium heat, warm the oil. Cook the onion, fennel, and garlic, stirring, for 5 to 7 minutes, or until the mixture is tender and translucent.

2. Increase the heat to high, add the beans and water, and bring to a boil. Reduce the heat to low, cover, and simmer for 2 hours, or until the beans are very tender. If using canned beans, cook, uncovered, for 30 minutes, or until the water is reduced and the soup has thickened.

3. Stir in the corn and tomatoes and cook for 5 minutes. Add the pepper, salt, and dill at the last minute. Serve warm or chilled.

succotash is a dish combining corn, beans (usually lima beans), bell peppers (optional), and lard or butter. It became very popular during the Great Depression due to its cheap, accessible ingredients and the satiating quality of the beans. My version uses olive oil, rich in omega-3 and omega-6 fatty acids, instead of animal-based fats.

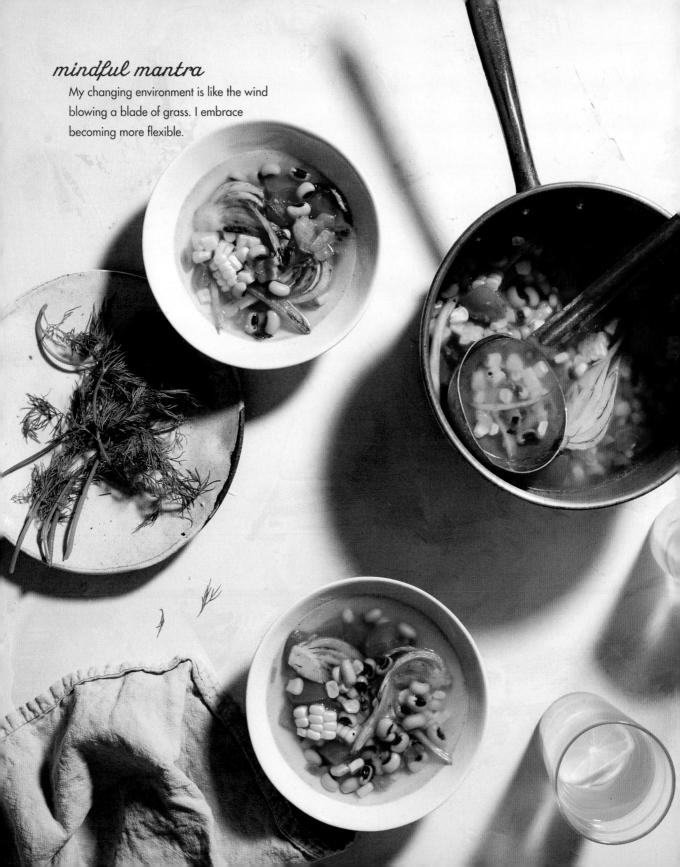

mindful mantra

My changing environment is like the wind blowing a blade of grass. I embrace becoming more flexible.

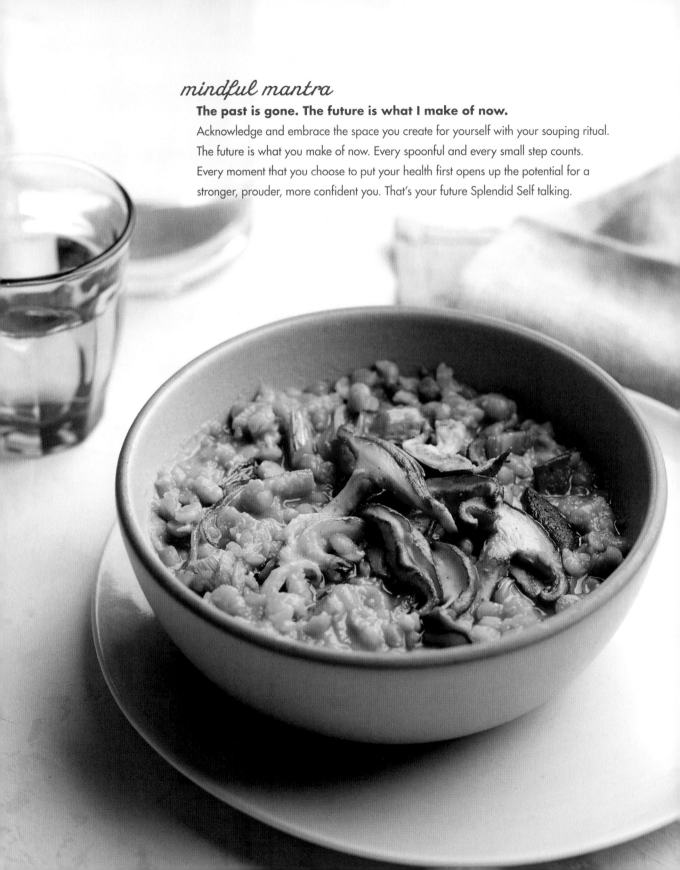

mindful mantra

The past is gone. The future is what I make of now.

Acknowledge and embrace the space you create for yourself with your souping ritual. The future is what you make of now. Every spoonful and every small step counts. Every moment that you choose to put your health first opens up the potential for a stronger, prouder, more confident you. That's your future Splendid Self talking.

SPLIT PEA *with* SHIITAKE "BACON"

1 cup shiitake caps, sliced into thin pieces

2 tablespoons olive oil, divided

1 small onion, diced

1 large clove garlic, minced

1 large carrot, diced (cut bigger chunks if you want the carrot to be more al dente in your finished soup)

1 rib celery, diced (cut bigger chunks if you want the celery to be more al dente in your finished soup)

½ teaspoon ground black pepper

2–3 sprigs fresh thyme, stems removed

2 teaspoons sea salt

½ pound dried split green or yellow peas

2 quarts water

1. Preheat the oven to 425°F.

2. On a baking sheet, toss the mushrooms with 1 tablespoon of the oil and spread into a single layer. Roast for 30 minutes, turning halfway through, or until the mushrooms are deep brown and a little chewy (but not burned!).

3. In a medium pot over medium heat, warm the remaining 1 tablespoon oil. Cook the onion, garlic, carrot, and celery, stirring frequently, for 5 to 10 minutes, or until soft and fragrant.

4. Increase the heat to medium-high. Stir in the pepper, thyme, salt, peas, and water and simmer, stirring occasionally, for 45 minutes, or until the peas fall apart completely.

5. Enjoy warm and garnish with the shiitake mushroom bacon. Store the shiitake bacon separately in an airtight container in the refrigerator if saving for later.

■ STRENGTHEN
■ MOM AND BABY

I bet you didn't think bacon would be a part of this Soup Cleanse. You thought right. Thanks to the earthy, meaty magic of shiitakes and the heat of your oven, this split pea soup is elevated to another level in flavor and savoriness. Roasting shiitake mushroom slices until they are a little chewy produces a remarkably bacon-like flavor.

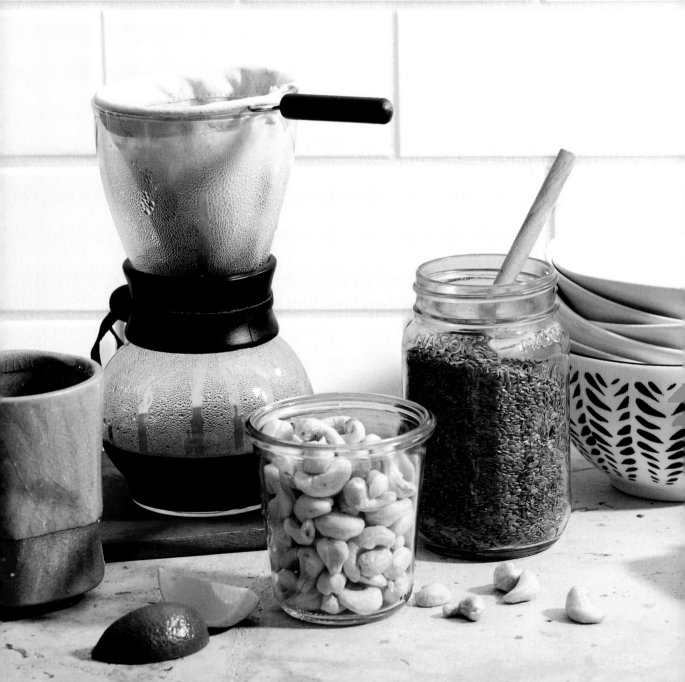

chapter 7

SWEETER

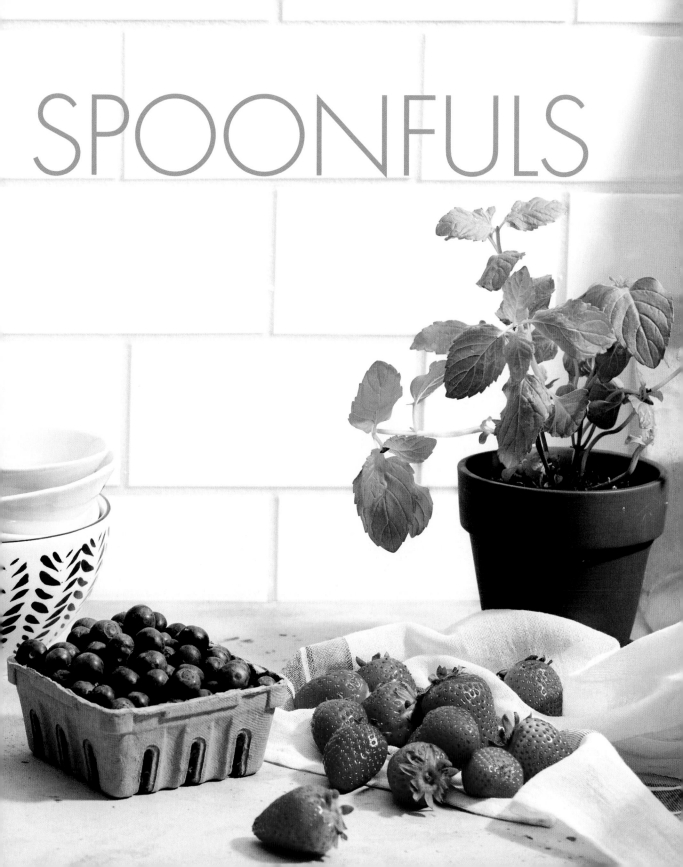

SPOONFULS

sweet soup? isn't that just a smoothie or a juice?

Splendid Spoon soups are full of fiber and focus on lower-sugar fruits (tomatoes and avocados are fruits, after all). A sweet tooth is nothing to shy away from in this case because I use warming seasonings, like cinnamon and nutmeg, to create sweeter profiles. The sugar content of these sweeter soups remains very low (less than 6 grams per bowl), especially in comparison to the plethora of sweet treats out there. We also call on nuts and seeds for support as they provide ample nutritional value in the form of protein and fat while helping to impart a sweeter taste. I also don't go full-on sweet for sweet's sake. Unsweetened cocoa, vanilla, and matcha create new angles from which you can experience a soup that sits somewhere between sweet and savory.

PUMPKIN APPLE

■ ENERGIZE
■ HEAL

4   pounds pumpkin, cut into 2" chunks, or 1 can (29 ounces)
    pumpkin puree (see note)

1   tablespoon coconut oil

2   apples, peeled and chopped into bite-size pieces (about 4 cups)

2   tablespoons grated fresh ginger

1   tablespoon finely chopped fresh sage

½   teaspoon ground red pepper (add more or less depending on
    your love of heat!)

    Sea salt and ground black pepper, to taste

1   cup water

1   cup apple cider (2 cups if using canned pumpkin)

1. Place a steamer basket in a large pot with 2" of water. Bring to a boil over high heat. Steam the pumpkin in the basket for 50 minutes, or until the pumpkin is tender and easily pierced with a knife. Skip this step if using canned pumpkin and add the pumpkin in Step 2.

2. Meanwhile, in a large pot over medium-high heat, warm the oil. Cook the apples, ginger, sage, red pepper, salt, and black pepper, stirring frequently, for 10 minutes, or until fragrant. Stir in the water and cook for 10 minutes, or until the apples are soft.

3. In a countertop blender, combine the cooked pumpkin or puree and the apple cider. Blend until smooth. Gently incorporate the pumpkin mixture into the apple mixture. Reduce the heat to low and warm the mixture.

4. Serve hot!

Note: The weight of a can of pumpkin puree is less than that of the fresh pumpkin called for because it has already been cooked down substantially. A 29-ounce can probably started with more like 4 to 5 pounds of fresh pumpkin.

Pumpkin mania sets in around September when the days start to get shorter and the air feels a little crisper. The hazy heavy days of summer are finally abating, and we all start to just *really* want to wear sweaters and eat things that taste like fall. And pumpkins are what fall tastes like, at least here in the Northeast. Ginger, sage, and ground red pepper are great team players in this soup as they add some sharper edges to pumpkin's rich flavor.

A NOTE ON STEAMING

Steaming vegetables is a really nice way to retain their nutrient value and color. Steam is a really efficient heat source, so you can cook a little quicker than with roasting, and the resulting flavor is a little cleaner. Personally, I love roasting because I think vegan recipes benefit from the deeper flavors achieved with roasting in fat. But a steamed vegetable has its own lovely appeal in its pared-down purity. You can steam in the microwave or on the stove top with a steamer pot, like I do here. If you don't have a steamer pot, you can create your own with a large pot and a metal colander that rests inside the pot. You just don't want the veggies to be in the water; it's the steam from the water that provides the cooking magic, not the boiling water.

STRAWBERRY RHUBARB

1½ pounds rhubarb, sliced into ½" pieces

½ vanilla pod, split and insides scraped, or ¼ teaspoon vanilla paste or vanilla extract

2 teaspoons grated orange peel

1 tablespoon maple syrup (optional)

Pinch of freshly ground nutmeg

2 quarts water

1½ pounds strawberries, larger berries halved

½ cup loosely packed fresh basil, coarsely chopped

1. In a medium pot over medium heat, combine the rhubarb, vanilla, orange peel, maple syrup (if using), nutmeg, and water, cover, and simmer for 25 minutes, or until the rhubarb is very soft.

2. Add the strawberries and simmer for 10 minutes. Add the basil for the last 30 seconds of simmering.

3. Using an immersion blender, puree the soup until very smooth.

■ ENERGIZE
■ HEAL
■ WEIGHT LOSS
■ MOM AND BABY

This soup may be on the sweeter side, but rhubarb is technically a vegetable. The tart flavor traditionally pairs with sweet-tart strawberries, and this is a popular combination in summer pies. My parents' neighbor Peg makes at least a pie a week using berries and rhubarb grown in her backyard. They are amazing and totally not part of my Soup Cleanse Day of souping! (But I do like to have a piece on a summer Wander Day.) I included some signature seasonings from that pie in this chilled soup: cinnamon, nutmeg, and vanilla. But I replaced the white sugar with a touch of maple syrup. Sip this soup and enjoy 2 servings of fruit *and* vegetables in every bowlful.

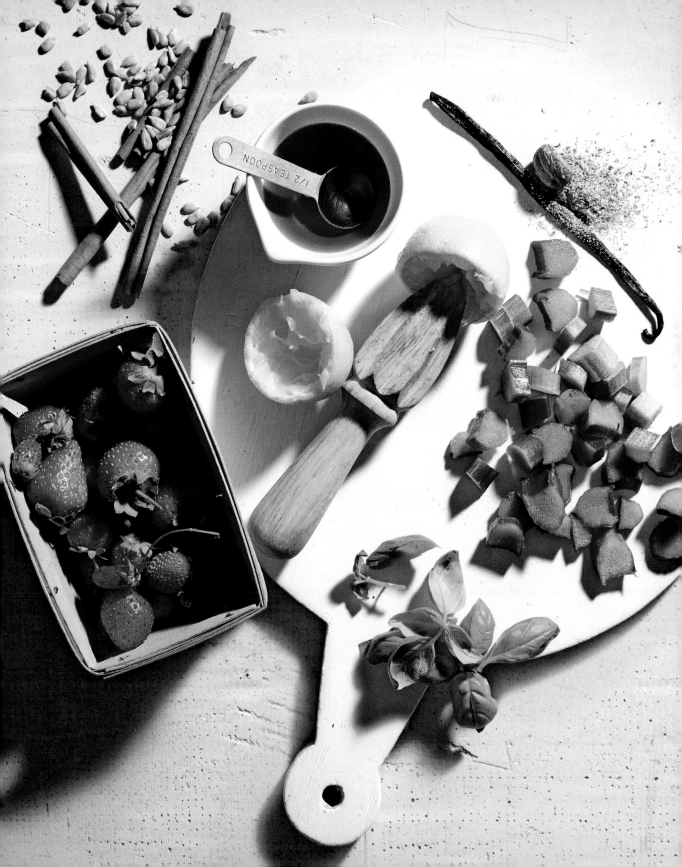

BERRY *and* FLAXSEED

■ ENERGIZE
■ HEAL
■ DETOX

- 1 quart plus ½ cup water
- 1 pound strawberries, quartered (about 3 cups)
- 6 ounces blueberries (about 2 cups)
- ¼ teaspoon finely chopped fresh thyme or ⅛ teaspoon dried
  Juice of 1 lime
- ¼ cup raw cashews, soaked overnight and drained (see "Why Soak Your Nuts and Seeds?" on page 74 for more information)
- ¼ cup ground flaxseed
  Peel of 1 lime, grated (about 2 teaspoons)
- ½ cup loosely packed fresh mint, torn

1. In a small pot over high heat, bring 1 quart of the water, the berries, and thyme to a boil. Reduce the heat to low and simmer for 40 minutes, or until the berries are soft and the liquid is reduced by half. Using the back of a mixing spoon, smash some of the berries about 15 minutes into cooking. Stir in the lime juice and take off the heat.

2. Meanwhile, in a countertop blender, combine the cashews, flaxseed, and the remaining ½ cup water and puree until very smooth. Swirl into the berry mixture. Top with the lime peel and mint.

When I was growing up, summer meant chasing my neighborhood friends through our suburban streets until sundown. We'd stop for snacks in each other's homes, begging parents for ice pops and ice cream sandwiches and mini bags of salty potato chips. When we'd exhausted the parents, we would literally root around in backyards and beside the bike path in town for other edibles. What we usually ended up with was berries, although sometimes we'd be brave enough to pull up the roots from the hardy native Queen Anne's lace flower and nibble on those. The roots of Queen Anne's lace—or wild carrots, as my mom called them—tasted like very tough parsnips and were more curiosity than summertime snack. The berries were perfection, though—tight and tart and sweet and warm—because by the time berries are in season, the sun is so hot you've forgotten what fall and winter ever felt like. This soup is wonderful chilled, but I like it right out of the pot because it reminds me of eating berries at twilight, their flesh still carrying the heat of the day.

CREAMY COCOA
with SWEET POTATOES

This soup is like a much cleaner version of rice pudding, and with a more sophisticated flavor. A bit of spice; a creamy bisquelike base of sweet potato, coconut, and cocoa; and flecks of tender black rice make this a soup you'll want to savor slowly.

1   large sweet potato, peeled and cut into 2" chunks (about 2 cups)

⅓   cup black rice

1   cup water

1   tablespoon 100% cocoa powder

    Pinch of ground red pepper

    Pinch of ground black pepper

½   teaspoon sea salt

1   can (15 ounces) coconut milk

1. Place a steamer basket in a large pot with 2" of water. Bring to a boil over high heat. Steam the sweet potato in the basket for 12 minutes, or until the potato is very soft and easily pierced with a knife. If you do not have a steamer basket, fill the pot with 1" of water and bring to a boil over high heat. Add the sweet potato. Reduce the heat to low, cover, and cook for about 10 minutes. Allow the potato to cool to room temperature. Reserve the water.

2. Meanwhile, in a medium pot over high heat, combine the rice and water, cover, and bring to a simmer. Reduce the heat to medium-low and cook for 40 minutes, or until the rice is tender.

3. In a countertop blender, combine the potatoes, the reserved steaming water, cocoa powder, red pepper, black pepper, salt, and coconut milk. Puree to a smoothie consistency.

4. Stir in the black rice. Enjoy warm or chilled.

cocoa beans are one of my favorite sources for flavonoids—uniquely plant-based compounds that have antioxidant properties. Not only is cocoa great for your health, but it also adds depth of flavor and beautiful color to this soup. It's said to release endorphins in your brain, too, which may be why we consider it an aphrodisiac. You can call it love, lust, or just pure joy, but we're always excited when this ingredient plays nicely with some of our vegetable friends.

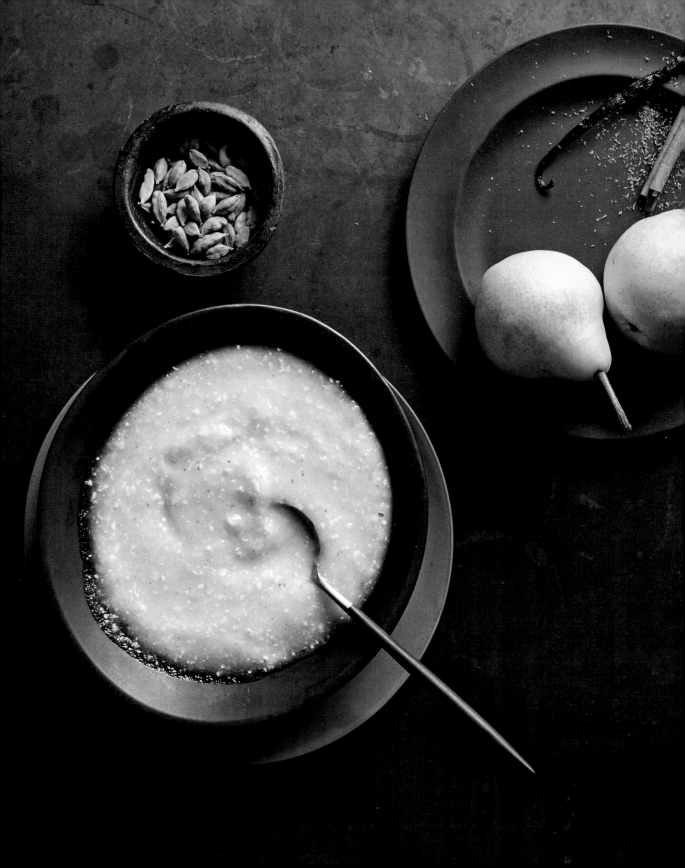

PEAR *and* SUNFLOWER SEED

2 pounds Bartlett pears, quartered

½ teaspoon freshly ground cardamom seeds or ¼ teaspoon dried

1 vanilla pod, split and insides scraped, or ½ teaspoon vanilla paste or vanilla extract

1 teaspoon ground Saigon cinnamon or conventional cinnamon

¼ cup sunflower seeds, soaked overnight and drained (see "Why Soak Your Nuts and Seeds?" on page 74 for more information)

1 tablespoon ground hempseed

Juice of ½ lemon

2 quarts water

1. In a medium pot over high heat, combine the pears, cardamom, vanilla, cinnamon, sunflower seeds, hempseed, lemon juice, and water, cover, and bring to a simmer.

2. Reduce the heat to low and simmer for 30 minutes, or until the pears are very soft.

3. Using an immersion blender or countertop blender, puree the soup until very smooth.

■ WEIGHT LOSS
■ DETOX

We use Bartlett pears from Fishkill Farms in Hopewell Junction, New York, when we make this soup at our microsoupery. Since this is a pureed soup, we happily take some of the more banged-up pears. If you offer to do the same at your local farmers' market, the farmer will probably give you a few extra pieces. The Bartlett variety has a very thin skin, which makes preparation that much easier (hooray, no peeling!), plus it gives you an extra dose of insoluble fiber to slow down sugar absorption.

HONEYDEW WITH MATCHA *and* MINT

■ **HEAL**
■ **WEIGHT LOSS**
■ **DETOX**

1   tablespoon matcha powder

¼   cup boiled water

½   honeydew melon, cut into 1" chunks (about 4 cups)

12 ounces coconut water

¼   cup shredded coconut

½   cup loosely packed fresh mint

½   cup loosely packed fresh basil

1. In a small bowl, whisk the matcha powder into the water to dissolve.

2. In a countertop blender, combine the tea, melon, coconut water, coconut, mint, and basil. Puree to a smoothie consistency.

3. Pour over ice.

Honeydew can be an incredibly juicy and sweet melon, and I encourage you to find the sweetest, juiciest one you can. A ripe melon will be unmistakably fragrant with a heavy, sweet aroma when you press its little belly button and then put your nose to it. The sweetness of the melon is tempered by the bitter herbal flavor of the matcha when these two green ingredients are combined. Plus, matcha boosts the antioxidant value significantly. Shredded coconut adds an extra element of delectableness to this soup; the sweet and fatty crumbles are nothing short of divine to chew on between sips.

there are books written on matcha. Very simply, it is a fine green powder made from the young green leaves of tea plants, traditionally grown and harvested in Japan. Depending on when the leaves are harvested and how finely they are ground, you will achieve different textures and flavors. A vibrant Technicolor green indicates a high-quality matcha. Dull green, not so much. My friends at Panatea create a beautiful matcha that's available online and ships nationally. In addition to using it in recipes, you can, of course, whisk it into a paste and then add more hot water to produce a cup of green tea. The flavor of a high-quality matcha will have a little bitterness that hits the back sides of your tongue and then rolls off into a gentle and fresh grassy flavor.

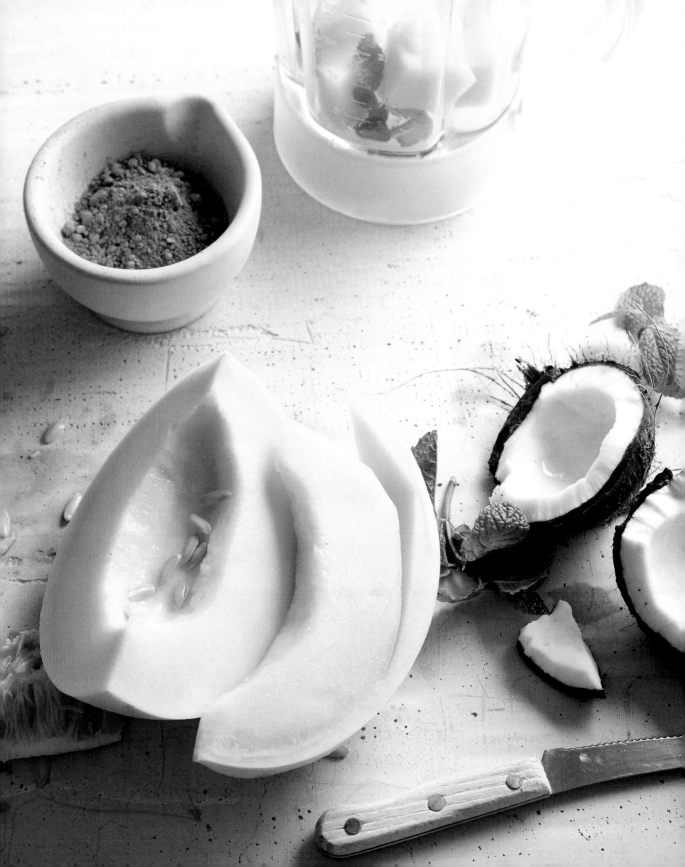

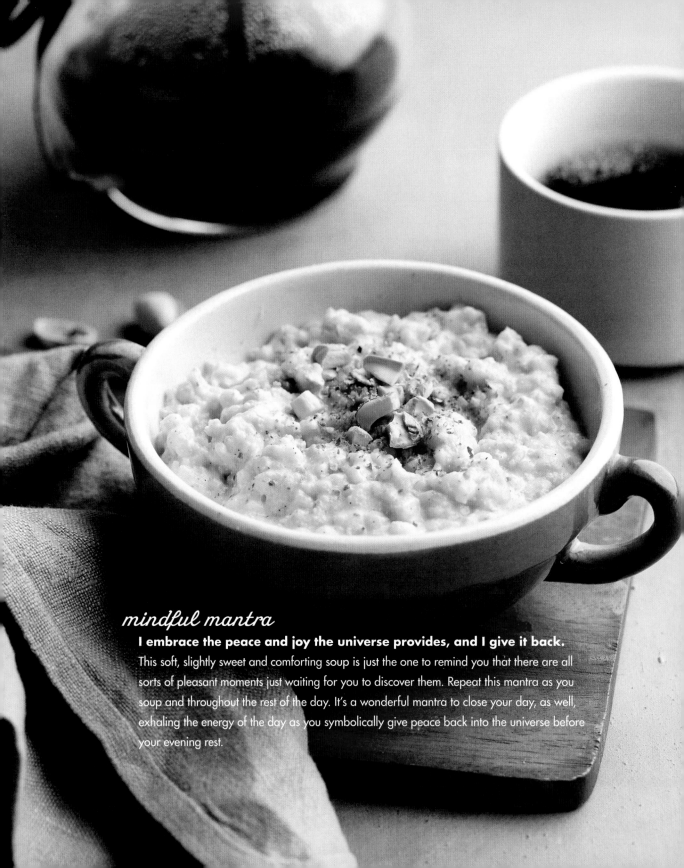

mindful mantra

I embrace the peace and joy the universe provides, and I give it back.

This soft, slightly sweet and comforting soup is just the one to remind you that there are all sorts of pleasant moments just waiting for you to discover them. Repeat this mantra as you soup and throughout the rest of the day. It's a wonderful mantra to close your day, as well, exhaling the energy of the day as you symbolically give peace back into the universe before your evening rest.

VANILLA PISTACHIO
with OATS

1½ quarts water

Pinch of sea salt

⅓ cup steel-cut oats

½ cup unsalted, roasted pistachios, shelled, soaked overnight, and drained (see "Why Soak Your Nuts and Seeds?" on page 74 for more information)

1 vanilla pod, split and insides scraped, or 1 teaspoon vanilla extract or paste

1 teaspoon ground cinnamon

Grated peel and juice of 1 large navel orange

1. In a large pot over high heat, bring the water to a boil. Add the salt and oats. Reduce the heat to low and simmer, stirring occasionally, for 30 minutes, or until the oats are very tender and creamy.

2. Meanwhile, in a countertop blender, puree the pistachios until very smooth. Pour into a small bowl and set aside. (Don't bother washing out the blender—you're about to use it again.)

3. Once the oats have cooked, stir in the vanilla and cinnamon. Place the mixture in the blender and puree until smooth.

4. Stir in the pistachio "milk," orange peel, and orange juice.

■ ENERGIZE
■ WEIGHT LOSS

This soup is more porridge than soup, and the steel-cut oats provide a superbly satisfying stage for the delicate flavors of orange, vanilla, and cinnamon to dance on. It's also surprisingly low in sugar for its sweet flavor. The vitamin E–rich pistachios and vanilla bean are what fool your taste buds, and you won't mind this kind of trickery!

vanilla beans have been used as a medicinal food for centuries, with claims of mood-enhancing powers. It seems these claims hold some weight as vanilla is a good source for magnesium, which plays an important role in regulating the nervous system.

GRAPEFRUIT *and* FENNEL CONSOMMÉ

1   tablespoon olive oil

1   small bulb fennel, thinly sliced (about 4 cups)

    Sea salt and ground black pepper, to taste

4   red grapefruits, segmented and chopped into bite-size pieces and juice reserved (about 4 cups flesh and 1 cup juice)

1   teaspoon grated orange peel

1   cup water

2   tablespoons chopped fresh dill

1. In a medium skillet over medium heat, warm the oil. Cook the fennel, salt, and pepper, stirring frequently, for 8 minutes, or until the fennel starts to caramelize. Add a splash of water and allow the steam to cook the fennel for 1 minute.

2. In a large bowl, combine the fennel, grapefruit juice and segments, orange peel, water, and dill.

3. Ladle into bowls and chill in the refrigerator for 1 hour or overnight. Enjoy chilled.

HOW TO SEGMENT CITRUS

This is one of my favorite kitchen skills since it creates that stained-glass segment of citrus: jewel-colored and free of white stringy pith. Slice off each pole of the grapefruit (this technique works for any citrus you might be segmenting), and stand the grapefruit lengthwise. Starting from the top pole, carve the peel off the grapefruit, curving the knife around the flesh and stopping when your knife hits the cutting board. Continue until all the peel is removed. Hold the nude little sphere of citrus in your palm over a bowl, and use your knife to cut the segments out of the pith until you have a bowl full of segments and a hand full of juicy pith. Squeeze every delicious ruby drop out of your grapefruit and over the segments. Discard the pith and peel.

This soup is like a tonic with the sweet and bitter grapefruit and potent licorice-like flavor of the fennel. Citrus and fennel both help your detox systems work smoother, and I think the fresh aroma of this soup has energizing and healing properties before you even taste that first spoonful. Enjoy the full sensory experience of this soup. It's prettier and more delicate than just about any other soup I make.

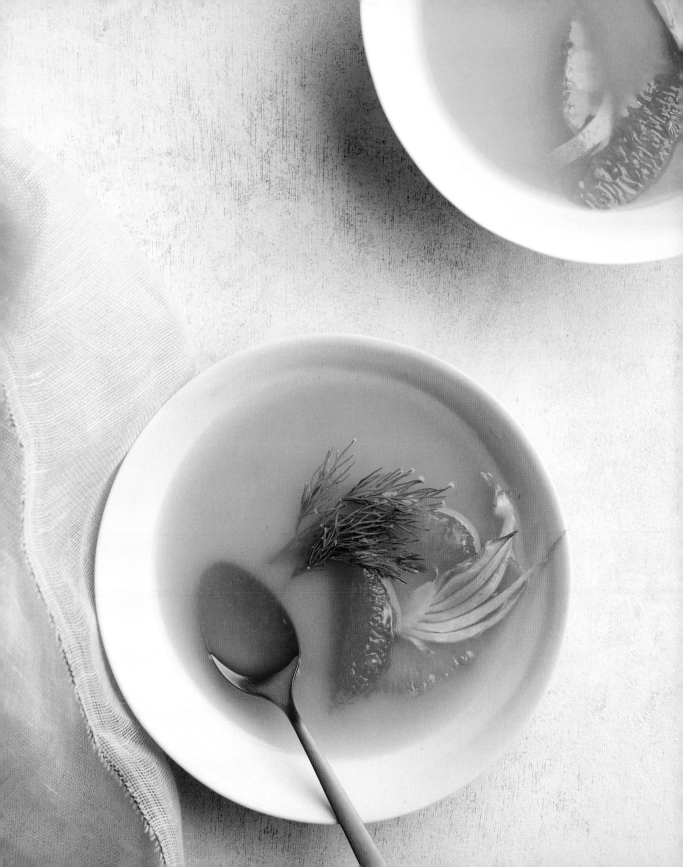

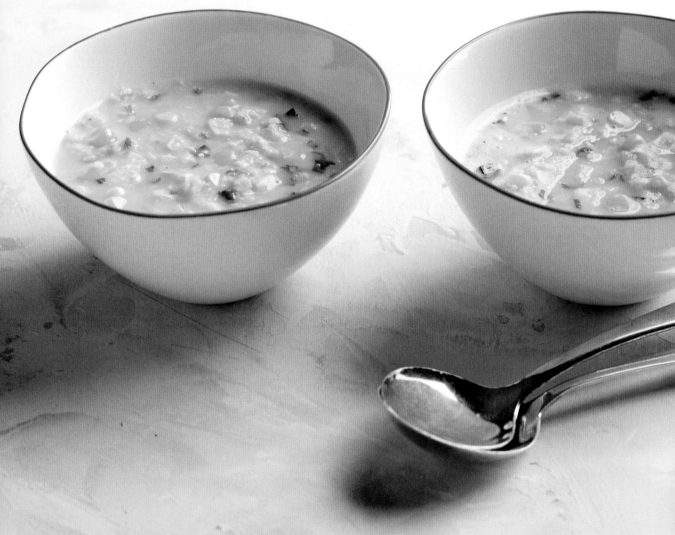

mindful movement

I challenge you to push a little bit!

Sign up for at least one more group activity than you typically participate in on a weekly basis: walking club, yoga class, any activity in a group setting. Moving with a group isn't just fun; it helps you establish a deeper connection to the action because you're getting an immediate reward from the social interaction. Recognize those good feelings, and remember that this healthy challenge is probably achievable with a few days' notice and a call or text message.

RAW NATIVE CORN
with BASIL

■ ENERGIZE
■ HEAL
■ DETOX
■ MOM AND BABY

2 quarts water

3 ears corn, kernels sliced off and cobs halved (about 3 cups kernels)

½ teaspoon sea salt

1 teaspoon olive oil

1 bunch scallions, white and pale green parts only, chopped (about 3 cups)

1 cup loosely packed fresh basil, torn

½ cup loosely packed fresh cilantro

1. In a medium pot over high heat, bring the water, corn cobs, and salt to a boil. Reduce the heat to low and simmer for about 15 minutes. Discard the cobs.

2. Meanwhile, in a skillet over medium heat, warm the oil. Cook the scallions for 3 minutes, or until they are soft.

3. In a countertop blender, combine the scallions, corn kernels, and half of the corn broth. Pulse to combine. Add the basil and cilantro and pulse to combine, adding more broth if necessary. (The soup should remain chunky.)

4. Serve warm or chilled.

This soup started as a vegan corn chowder and transformed into the epitome of a truly refreshing, chilled summer treat. The basil and cilantro are abundant at the same time of year as the corn, and you can measure in handfuls instead of cups if you are trying to use a little more of these delicate herbs lest you miss out on their summer growing season. (Or perhaps they've overrun your garden like they do to my Mom's every July.) Choose the freshest picked corn you can get your hands on, and put a friend or little one to work husking while you sauté the scallions.

corn gets a bad rap for being genetically modified (GMO). However, if you are getting your corn from a small farm, most likely you are safe. If you are really concerned about contamination from other GMO farms in your area, you could politely ask the farmer whether he thinks his crop is at risk for seed drift. Native corn is delightfully sweet in flavor and high in insoluble fiber and vitamin C. Since this is a barely cooked soup, that vitamin C (a vitamin that is sensitive to heat) stays intact.

MINTY MELON CHIA

■ HEAL
■ WEIGHT LOSS
■ DETOX

1   seedless watermelon, diced and divided (about 6 cups)

¼   cup ground chia seeds

     Sea salt and ground black pepper, to taste

2   tablespoons grated fresh ginger

     Peel of 1 lemon, grated (about 2 teaspoons)

     Juice of 1 lemon

1   cup water

1   cup loosely packed fresh mint, sliced in a chiffonade
     and divided (see "Chiffo-What? Chiffonade!"
     for how to chiffonade)

This cooling soup is fun to make with kids because it doesn't require cooking—and, come on, who doesn't love watermelon in the summer? A little ginger, a lot of mint, and chia seeds give this chilled soup a more grown-up flavor. Plus the chia seeds boost the nutritional value with all their protein.

1. In a countertop blender, combine half of the watermelon, the chia seeds, salt, pepper, ginger, lemon peel, lemon juice, water, and half of the mint. Puree until smooth.

2. Divide the remaining watermelon into 4 bowls. Spoon the blended watermelon mixture into each bowl. Sprinkle the remaining mint on top.

CHIFFO-WHAT? CHIFFONADE!

This technique sounds fancy, but I like it because I think it makes slicing fresh herbs easier. It works best with broader-leaf herbs like the mint in this recipe, as well as basil or sage. Simply pluck your leaves from the stem, stack them (make a few stacks if you have a lot of leaves, like you will in this recipe), and then roll tightly to form a teeny roll. Take your knife and slice through the roll crosswise from end to end. You'll be left with a little crumpled pile of herbs. Fluff them and you'll see the rolled-up pieces unravel into longer ribbons. If you keep your slices close together, the resulting herb ribbons will be light and thin. Easy, right? Chiffo-nod your head yes.

everyone loves talking about chia as a secret superfood from Central and South America. It's a little itty-bitty seed that swells and becomes gelatinous when mixed with water. It's special because of its mix of omega-3 and omega-6 fatty acids and because it's a very efficient source of protein (5 grams in just 1 teaspoon), but the best way for your body to access chia fat and protein is to grind those seeds first. Similar to flaxseed, your body simply cannot break through the tough outer shell of chia, and you'll be doing yourself a big favor by buying ground chia or grinding it yourself.

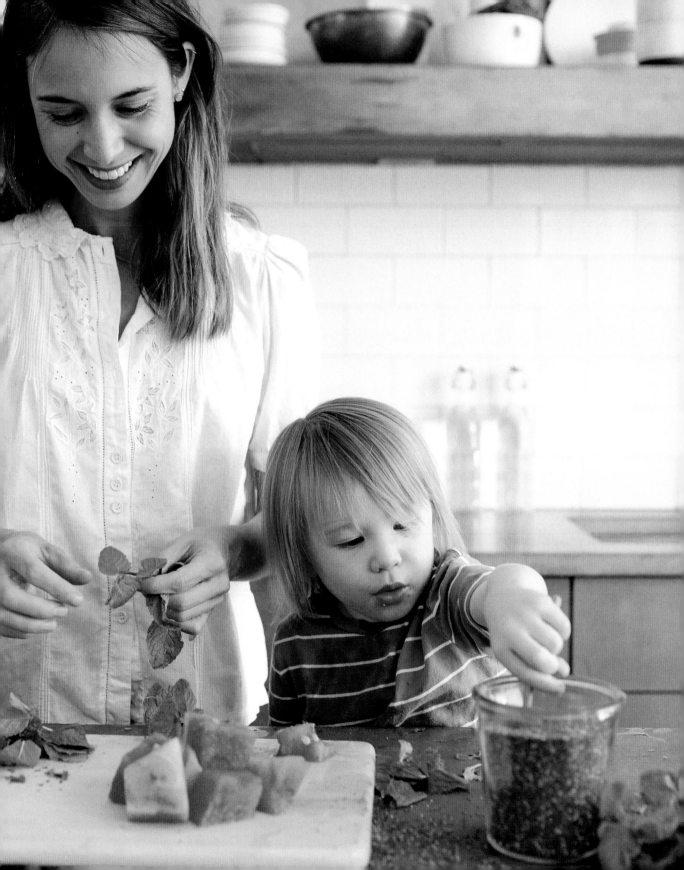

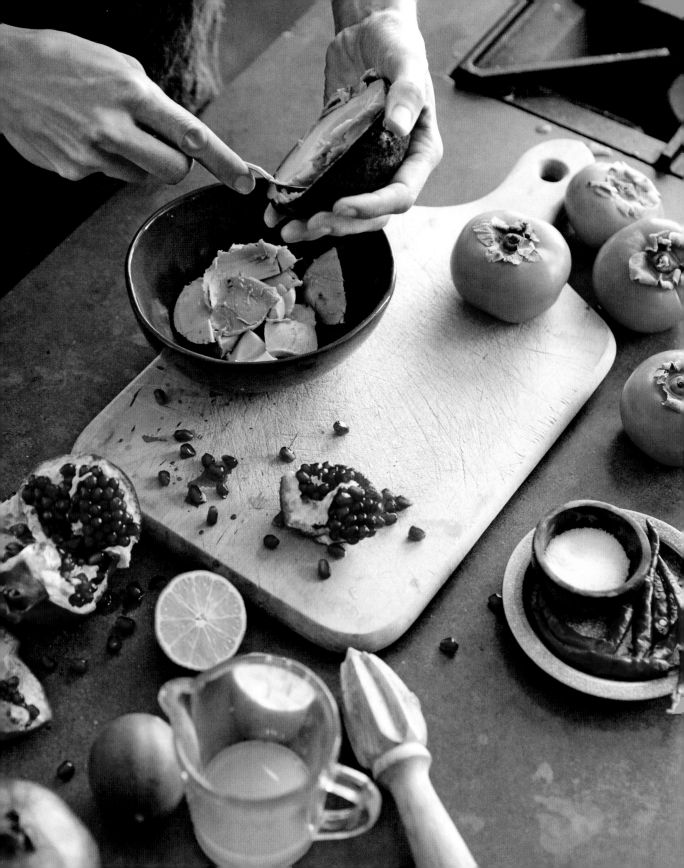

SWEET POTATO SOUP WITH PERSIMMONS *and* POMEGRANATE

■ HEAL
■ WEIGHT LOSS
■ DETOX

Persimmon and pomegranate come into season in late November. While we import them in the Northeast, they still carry a festive seasonal aspect that signals the coming of Thanksgiving and Christmas. This soup combines roasted sweet potatoes and persimmons with raw pomegranate so you get every drop of vitamin C these punchy seeds have to offer. That's a great thing because as the weather turns colder, our immune systems need an extra boost to adjust to the changing air pressure and moisture and the different bugs that like to live in this new environment. I finish this pretty orange soup with bright lime and a smushy spoonful of avocado.

- 2 large sweet potatoes, peeled and diced
- 3 very ripe Fuyu persimmons, chopped into ½" pieces (about 2 cups)
- 2 tablespoons olive oil
  Peel of 2 limes, grated (about 4 teaspoons)
  Juice of 2 limes
  Pinch of sea salt
- ½ jalapeño pepper, seeds removed, finely chopped (use gloves if your skin is sensitive to hot peppers)
- 1 quart water
- 1 cup pomegranate seeds
- ½ avocado, mashed (optional)

1. Preheat the oven to 425°F.
2. On a baking sheet, toss the sweet potatoes and persimmons together with the oil and spread into a single layer. Cover with foil and roast for 20 minutes. Remove the foil and roast for 15 minutes.
3. In a countertop blender, combine the roasted potatoes and persimmons, lime peel, lime juice, salt, and jalapeño pepper. Blend, adding the water gradually to achieve a milk-shake consistency. (It may not be necessary to add all the water.)
4. Mound a quarter of the pomegranate seeds into each of 4 bowls and pour the orange soup around the seeds. This soup is lovely at room temperature, heated a little more, or even chilled. I like a spoonful of mashed avocado swirled in, too.

fuyus are my favorite to work with because Hachiyas are unpalatably tart unless perfectly ripe. Fuyus have a mildly sweet flavor reminiscent of papaya. To prepare, peel with a vegetable peeler, cut out the core, and chop.

a mindful moment

with your pomegranates

I have a special appreciation for pomegranates because of their association with the birth of my second son, Caleb. I woke up around 3 a.m. knowing I would be going into labor within the next 24 hours. I was uncomfortable and starting to feel contractions but knew I didn't need to call my midwife yet or start getting ready for the trip to the hospital. Caleb was born on December 7, right in the middle of pomegranate season, and I had a beautiful mound of the ripe red globes in a bowl on my counter, like a bowlful of Christmas ornaments. From 3 a.m. until whenever the first light started to show, I slowly opened those pomegranates and took out the seeds. It was meditative for me to gently pull out the translucent jewels (or arils, as the edible seeds are called). I felt like I was doing my part to prepare something sweet for my older son, Grover, to enjoy while I was away. Plus it was helpful to focus on this peaceful task as my body progressed with contractions—that was the meditative element. So every time I open a pomegranate, I slow down and really appreciate the time it takes to free those sweet seeds. My way: I slice the pomegranate in half (you will see the seeds clustered together in little bunches with thin, papery pith dividing the clusters) and gently peel it open a bit so I can get my thumb tips around a few seeds at a time and gently roll them out, focusing on one cluster at a time. I do this over a bowl or resealable container so they are easy to cover and put into the fridge for storage. Another option is to hold the pomegranate half so it is skin side up and whack the back with a wooden spoon. The seeds will shake out into a large bowl before you. I could see this being cathartic or meditative for all sorts of reasons, but I'm more the slow, methodical type when it comes to pomegranates.

SPICED FIG *and* CASHEW

½ cup cashews

6 cups water, divided

1 pound fresh figs or 2½ cups dried, halved

½ cup dried dates, halved

½ teaspoon ground cloves

½ teaspoon ground ginger

½ teaspoon ground cinnamon

Grated peel and juice from 1 orange

1. In a medium saucepan over high heat, bring the cashews, 3 cups of the water, figs, dates, cloves, ginger, and cinnamon to a boil. Reduce the heat to low, cover, and simmer for 30 minutes, or until the cashews are soft and the dates (and dried figs, if using) are hydrated.

2. In a countertop blender, combine the remaining 3 cups water, the cashew mixture, orange peel, and orange juice and puree until very smooth (the consistency of a thin milk shake).

3. Enjoy warm or chilled.

■ ENERGIZE
■ DETOX
■ WEIGHT LOSS
■ MOM AND BABY

This creamy soup is like a chai latte without all the sugar. This is probably the sweetest of the bunch, but the clove, ginger, and grated orange peel keep it from getting annoying. This soup is awesome with dried figs and totally divine with fresh ones. The cashew milk holds it all together and adds the right amount of protein and fat to balance the natural sugars of the fruit and keep your body from digesting them too quickly.

ROASTED CHESTNUTS
with SAIGON CINNAMON

2 pounds chestnuts in shell, scored, or 4 cups jarred chestnuts

1 tablespoon olive oil

1 small onion, diced

1 large apple, any variety, diced (about 2 cups)

2 ribs celery, diced

1 clove garlic, minced

2 teaspoons Saigon cinnamon or conventional cinnamon

Pinch of ground red pepper (optional)

1 quart water

½ teaspoon sea salt

Just like pumpkins scream fall, chestnuts ring in winter. Chestnuts are tree nuts that are native to the Northeast and provide a healthy dose of fiber, protein, and B-complex vitamins that help boost brain function. Swap out your mug of eggnog for this healthy soup that doubles as a very fragrant hand warmer.

1. Preheat the oven to 425°F.

2. Place the chestnuts in a single layer on a baking sheet and roast for 20 minutes, or until fragrant and the shells open. Remove from the oven and cover with a clean dish towel, allowing to steam for another 10 minutes. Peel the tough outer shells and cut into quarters. Make sure to peel the chestnuts while they are still warm or this task will be a challenge!

3. While the chestnuts are cooling, in a medium pot over medium heat, warm the oil. Cook the onion, apple, celery, and garlic, stirring frequently, for 5 to 10 minutes, or until the apples are tender and the onions are soft. Stir in the cinnamon, red pepper (if using), and quartered chestnuts and cook for 10 minutes, or until fragrant.

4. Add the water and salt. Increase the heat to high and bring to a boil. Reduce the heat and simmer for about 20 minutes, or until the chestnuts are very soft and the water is reduced.

5. Using an immersion blender, puree until very smooth (you want a thick consistency).

6. Sip warm from a mug!

chestnuts look much more intimidating than they are. The soft nut is encased in what looks like an impenetrable shell. It's actually fairly soft and can be easily pierced by a paring knife. The best way to roast chestnuts is to make a crisscross cut with a knife. The nut will expand as it roasts and you will be able to peel back the flexible outer shell to reveal the chestnut flesh after roasting. Don't forget to score those chestnuts; they make a hot and nearly impossible to clean mess if they explode (not that I would know or anything).

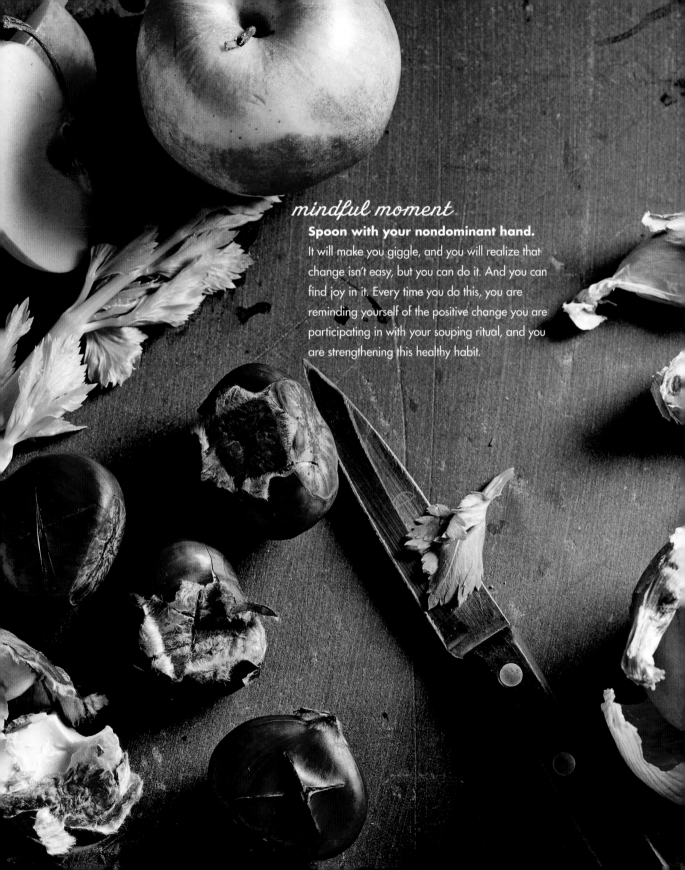

mindful moment

Spoon with your nondominant hand.
It will make you giggle, and you will realize that
change isn't easy, but you can do it. And you can
find joy in it. Every time you do this, you are
reminding yourself of the positive change you are
participating in with your souping ritual, and you
are strengthening this healthy habit.

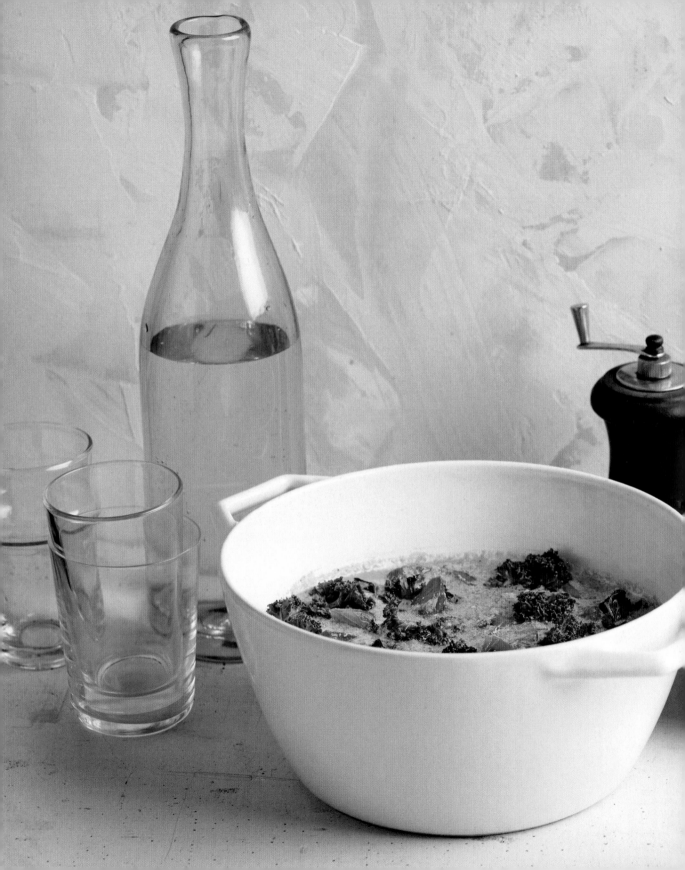

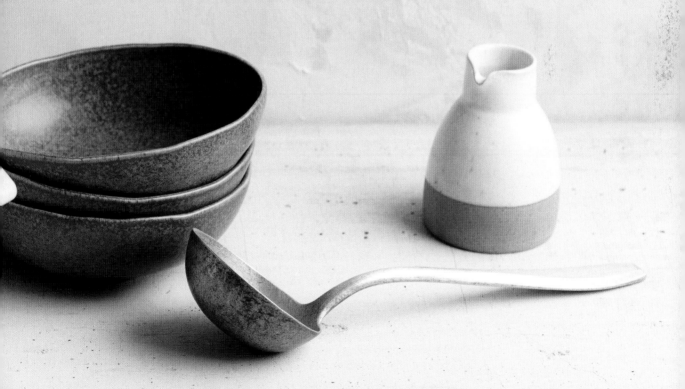

chapter 8

RESTORATIVE STEWS

stews are my favorite dinner. Splendid Spoon stews have a rich broth, lots of chunky vegetables, and ample opportunity for chewing. The stews are more complex in flavor than some of the other soups because they tend to have a few more ingredients. Traditionally, a stew was a type of leftover saver—combine the scraps of the kitchen in a pot and let it simmer together until it melds into one homogeneous mush. I go the other direction with stews, starting with fresh vegetables and a flavorful base rich with aromatic vegetables like onions and garlic, scallions and celery. Stews like to be layered, and you'll notice this in your souping experience as you eat. You'll remember that there was one more step in your stew versus making a broth and notice how different it tastes because of that. The layering of texture and flavor is what makes the stew so satisfying. That, and these are denser recipes with more vegetable content. So chew slowly and enjoy this meal in a bowl because there will likely be no leftovers from this pot.

SPICY BROCCOLI *and* HEMPSEED STEW

1½ quarts water

4 cups broccoli florets (bite-size pieces)

1 teaspoon coconut oil

2 scallions, sliced

1 cup dried chickpeas, soaked overnight and drained, or 1 can (15 ounces) low-sodium chickpeas, rinsed and drained

½ cup hempseed

1 teaspoon sea salt (omit if using canned beans)

½ teaspoon red-pepper flakes

Juice of 1 lime

Peel of 1 lime, grated (about 2 teaspoons)

1 tablespoon chopped fresh cilantro

1 tablespoon chopped fresh mint

1. Place a steamer basket in a large pot with 1 quart of the water. Bring to a boil over high heat. Steam the broccoli in the basket for 15 minutes, or until the broccoli is tender. (See "A Note on Steaming" on page 117 for more tips on steaming.) Reserve the steaming water.

2. In a medium pot over medium heat, warm the oil. Cook the scallions for 5 minutes, or until they are soft and translucent. Stir in the chickpeas, the water reserved from the steamed broccoli, and the remaining ½ quart water and cook for 1 hour (or 15 minutes for the canned chickpeas), or until the chickpeas are tender.

3. Stir in the hempseed, salt, red-pepper flakes, lime juice, and lime peel and cook for a few minutes. Using an immersion blender, puree the soup until smooth. Or puree the soup in a countertop blender and then add back to the pot.

4. Stir in the steamed broccoli, cilantro, and mint and cook on medium for 2 to 3 minutes just to reheat the broccoli.

5. Ladle into warm bowls.

■ ENERGIZE
■ STRENGTHEN
■ MOM AND BABY

I love this stew! The blended base gets its spice from simple red-pepper flakes, and the body comes from chickpeas, a reliable pantry basic in the Splendid Spoon kitchen—but there's nothing basic about this stew. Hempseed provides a complete set of amino acids to give your body every building block it needs to fuel the strengthening of its muscles. (And hopefully you're moving them more and more as you deepen your connection to souping and invite the mantras and movements into your daytime routine.) I really enjoy the fresh morsels of broccoli, but this flavor is easily transformed into a full-on puree. I've been known to puree the leftovers of this soup for a spicy breakfast. It's interesting how a change in texture can transform the whole experience of a soup, isn't it?

COURGETTE STEW

■ HEAL
■ WEIGHT LOSS
■ DETOX

2 tablespoons olive oil

1 large onion, diced

2 large cloves garlic, minced

1 tablespoon fresh thyme or 1 teaspoon dried

2 courgettes (aka yellow and green squash of any variety), chopped (about 3 cups)

Sea salt and ground black pepper, to taste

1 tablespoon tomato paste

1 quart water

2 pounds tomatoes, chopped, or 1 can (28 ounces) diced tomatoes

Lemon wedges for garnish (optional)

Get planted in this rich vegetable stew, teeming with yellow and green shades of summer zucchini and fresh aromatic thyme stewed in shimmering red tomatoes that burst with the energy of the sun.

1. In a large pot over medium heat, warm the oil. Cook the onion for 5 minutes, stirring occasionally, or until it is soft and translucent. Add the garlic and thyme and cook for 1 minute, or until fragrant.

2. Stir in the courgettes, salt, and pepper. Reduce the heat to medium-low and cook, stirring frequently, for 8 minutes, or until the courgettes are soft.

3. Stir in the tomato paste, water, and tomatoes. Increase the heat to high and bring to a boil. Reduce the heat to medium and simmer, uncovered, for 40 minutes, or until the mixture thickens.

4. Enjoy warm or chilled with the lemon wedges, if using.

is it zucchini? Is it squash? Yes and yes. Both belong to the family *Cucurbita pepo*. While squash originated in the Americas, zucchini—the long, green, cucumber-like plant—is a variety of squash that was developed in Italy several generations later.

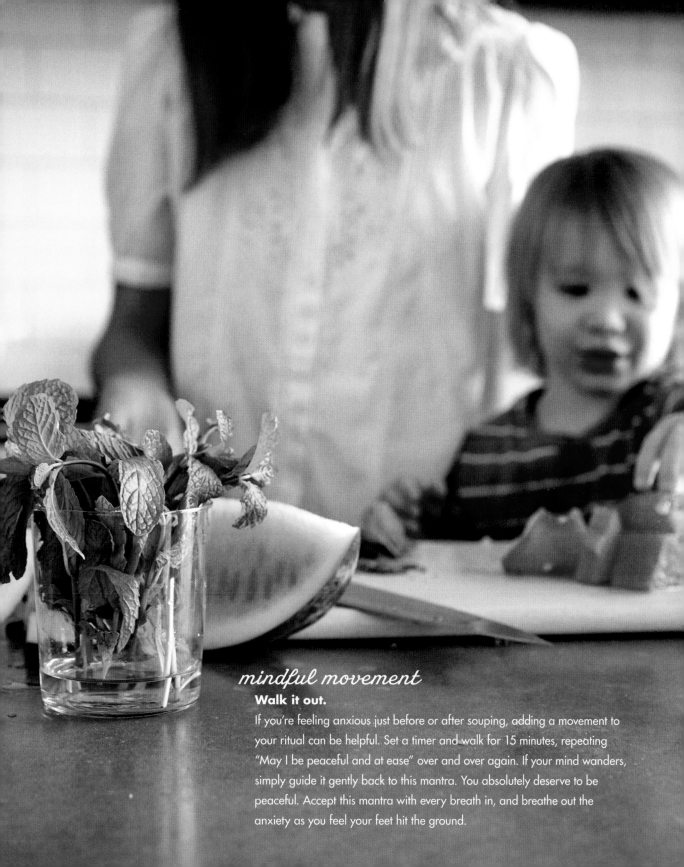

mindful movement

Walk it out.

If you're feeling anxious just before or after souping, adding a movement to your ritual can be helpful. Set a timer and walk for 15 minutes, repeating "May I be peaceful and at ease" over and over again. If your mind wanders, simply guide it gently back to this mantra. You absolutely deserve to be peaceful. Accept this mantra with every breath in, and breathe out the anxiety as you feel your feet hit the ground.

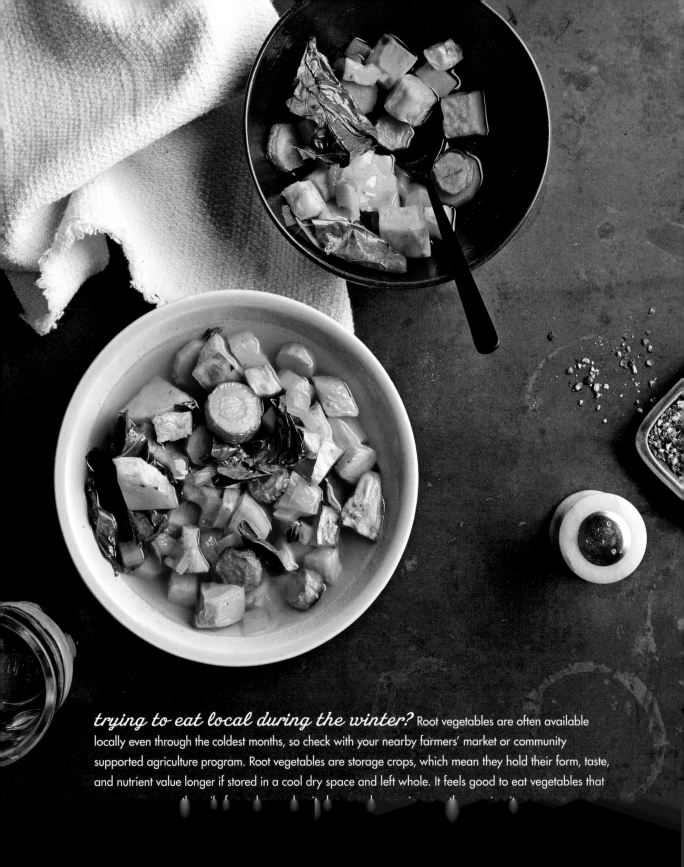

trying to eat local during the winter? Root vegetables are often available locally even through the coldest months, so check with your nearby farmers' market or community supported agriculture program. Root vegetables are storage crops, which mean they hold their form, taste, and nutrient value longer if stored in a cool dry space and left whole. It feels good to eat vegetables that

WINTER ROOT VEGETABLE STEW

1 small celeriac, peeled and diced (about 4 cups)

1 sweet potato, diced (about 2 cups)

2 carrots, diced

3 tablespoons olive oil, divided

1 yellow onion, diced

1 large clove garlic, chopped

2 tablespoons chopped fresh rosemary or ½ teaspoon dried

1 teaspoon sea salt

1 heaping teaspoon curry powder

½ teaspoon ground black pepper

1 quart homemade vegetable stock (such as the Vegan Bone Broth on page 174) or low-sodium store-bought broth

2 cups loosely packed collard greens, tough stems removed and leaves sliced in a chiffonade (see "Chiffo-What? Chiffonade!" on page 132 for a how-to of this technique)

1. Preheat the oven to 425°F.

2. On a baking sheet, toss the celeriac, sweet potato, and carrots with 2 tablespoons of the oil. Spread the vegetables in a single layer and cover with foil. Roast for 25 minutes. Remove the foil, toss the vegetables, and roast for 20 minutes, uncovered, or until the vegetables are tender when pierced with a fork.

3. In a medium pot over medium heat, warm the remaining 1 tablespoon oil. Cook the onion and garlic, stirring, for 7 to 10 minutes, or until the mixture is tender and translucent.

4. Stir in the rosemary, salt, curry powder, and pepper and cook for 2 to 3 minutes. Add the roasted vegetables and gently combine.

5. Add the stock or broth. Increase the heat to high and bring to a boil. Reduce the heat to medium, add the collard greens, cover, and simmer for about 10 minutes.

6. Ladle into warm bowls, drizzle with olive oil, and spoon slowly to savor every morsel!

■ ENERGIZE
■ HEAL
■ DETOX

Sweet potatoes come packed with vitamins A, B, C, and D; collard greens bring a bold dose of vitamin K for bone-building health, and rosemary's antifungal and anti-inflammatory components make it an herbal powerhouse. All the vegetables in this stew can be found in the winter even in more frigid climates. (Spinach too since it's grown more and more in greenhouses nationally!) I love this soup because even though the finished product reflects the more subdued palette of root vegetables, it feels fresh, light, and invigorating. It's grounding and uplifting all at once, which is just what I need on winter days when I don't get to play outside as much.

ANTIOXIDANT STEW

■ HEAL
■ DETOX

2 tablespoons olive oil

1 yellow onion, chopped

1 clove garlic, minced

1 tablespoon 100% cocoa powder

1 teaspoon sea salt

Pinch of ground black pepper

1 large beet, peeled and chopped (about 4 cups)

1 quart water

⅓ cup black rice or wild rice

1 cup dry red wine (see note)

With rich red wine, deep cocoa powder, and jewel-toned beets, this may be the most romantic of all my soups. I like using cocoa in savory dishes, and just a tablespoon goes a long way to add a grown-up bitter flavor and rich texture that complements the sweetness of the beets and the acidity of the red wine.

1. In a large pot over medium heat, warm the oil. Cook the onion for 3 to 5 minutes, or until it is soft and translucent. Stir in the garlic and cook for 2 minutes, or until fragrant.

2. Stir in the cocoa powder, salt, and pepper and cook for 1 minute. Add the beets and cook for 15 minutes, or until the beets are tender.

3. Add the water and stir to combine. Increase the heat to high and bring to a boil. Reduce the heat to medium-low, add the rice and wine, cover, and simmer for 35 minutes, or until the rice is soft but still has some bite to it (al dente).

4. Serve warm.

Note: The alcohol from the wine will cook off in Step 3, but the heart-healthy antioxidant resveratrol will remain.

similar to coffee, cocoa is an excellent source of antioxidants that trap cancer-causing free radicals. Much like how we consume coffee (with high amounts of animal fat and sugar to combat the bitterness), it's what we add to cocoa in the form of chocolate that can make it a "whoa" food instead of a "go" food. However, it's all go-time with cocoa's incarnation here.

CURLY KALE STEW

■ ENERGIZE
■ HEAL
■ WEIGHT LOSS
■ DETOX

2 tablespoons coconut oil

1 large onion, diced

3 cloves garlic, minced

1 teaspoon tomato paste

1 teaspoon sea salt

1 tablespoon Madras curry powder

½ teaspoon red-pepper flakes

2 cups chopped tomatoes or 1 can (14 ounces) crushed tomatoes

2 cups chopped curly kale

1 can (15 ounces) coconut milk

1 tablespoon grated fresh ginger

½ quart water plus more as needed

Everyone loves talking about Lacinato kale, also called dinosaur kale, because its deep green, pebbly leaves are so beautiful to look at. But curly kale has its merits, too. I prefer it in this stew because the curly parts of the kale embrace whatever comes near it, be it the coconut milk–laced broth, bits of ginger, or little flecks of hot pepper. Stews are such a welcome part of a soup cleanse because they really remind you that soup can be a varied textural experience, as well. Nothing like bits of spicy ginger or creamy coconut broth to surprise you in all the right ways.

1. In a large pot over medium heat, warm the oil. Cook the onion and garlic for 5 to 7 minutes, or until the mixture is soft and fragrant. Stir in the tomato paste, salt, curry, and red-pepper flakes and cook for 1 minute.

2. Add the tomatoes, kale, coconut milk, ginger, and ½ quart water. Increase the heat to high and bring to a boil. Reduce the heat to medium and simmer for 25 minutes, or until the mixture thickens and the kale is soft. Add more water if the soup is too thick.

3. Enjoy warm or chilled.

mindful mantra

My actions build confidence.

Confidence is a state of being, but our bodies can help us get there with movement. Reaching for a bowl, opening a drawer to find a spoon, sitting down—these are all movements toward rewarding habits. Don't brush that off! Acknowledge these actions and stand up taller as you perform them. Say this mantra to yourself through each movement from the beginning to the end of your souping ritual: My actions build confidence.

SUMMER RATATOUILLE

1   small eggplant, chopped into bite-size pieces (about 8 cups)

2   teaspoons sea salt, divided

2   tablespoons olive oil

1   onion, finely chopped

2   large cloves garlic, chopped

2   tablespoons finely chopped fresh oregano
    or 2 teaspoons dried

1   teaspoon red-pepper flakes (optional)

1   zucchini, diced (about 2 cups)

    Ground black pepper, to taste

2   tablespoons tomato paste

3   tomatoes (about 2 cups chopped) or 1 can (14 ounces)
    diced or crushed tomatoes

1   quart water

1   small head bok choy, green leaves only, thinly sliced
    (about 2 cups)

½   cup fresh basil, thinly sliced

Layers upon layers of summer-ripe flavor adorn every bite of this beautiful stew. Take full advantage of your local farmers' market to hunt down the freshest tomatoes, zucchini, and bok choy for your stew.

1. Place the eggplant in a strainer over a bowl. Toss with 1 teaspoon of the salt. Let sit while you prepare the other vegetables and cook the onion and garlic.

2. Meanwhile, in a large pot over medium heat, warm the oil. Cook the onion, garlic, oregano, and red-pepper flakes (if using), stirring, for 7 to 10 minutes, or until the mixture is soft and translucent. Turn off the heat.

3. Rinse the salted eggplant under running water and squeeze the cubes gently with your hands to remove as much moisture as possible.

4. In the same pot over medium heat, add the eggplant and zucchini. Season with the pepper and the remaining 1 teaspoon salt. Cook, stirring frequently, for 10 to 15 minutes, or until the eggplant and zucchini are soft.

5. Stir in the tomato paste, tomatoes, water, and bok choy. Increase the heat to high and bring to a boil. Reduce the heat to medium and simmer, uncovered, for 30 minutes, or until the mixture thickens and all the vegetables are very soft.

6. Serve warm or chilled with the basil sprinkled on top.

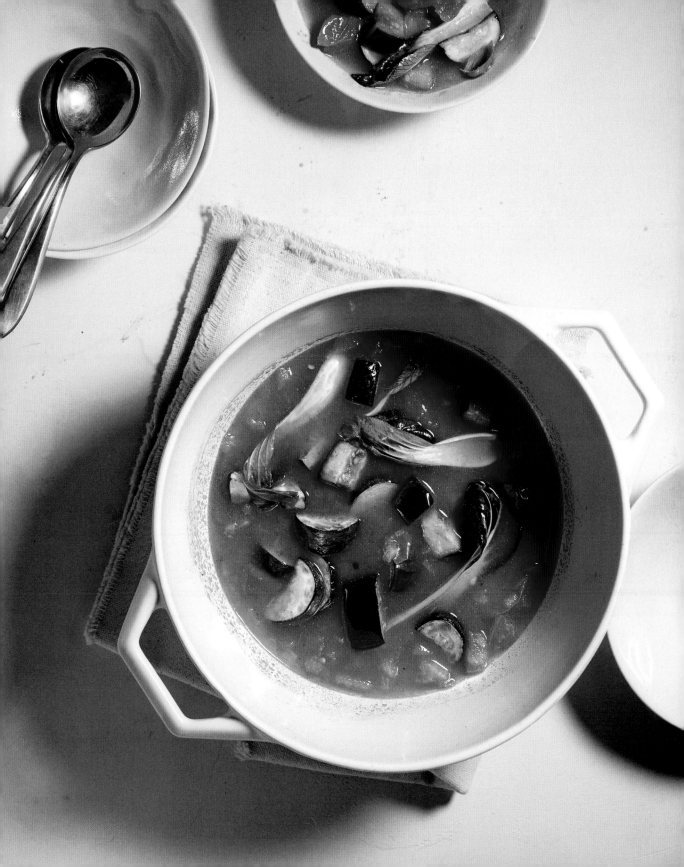

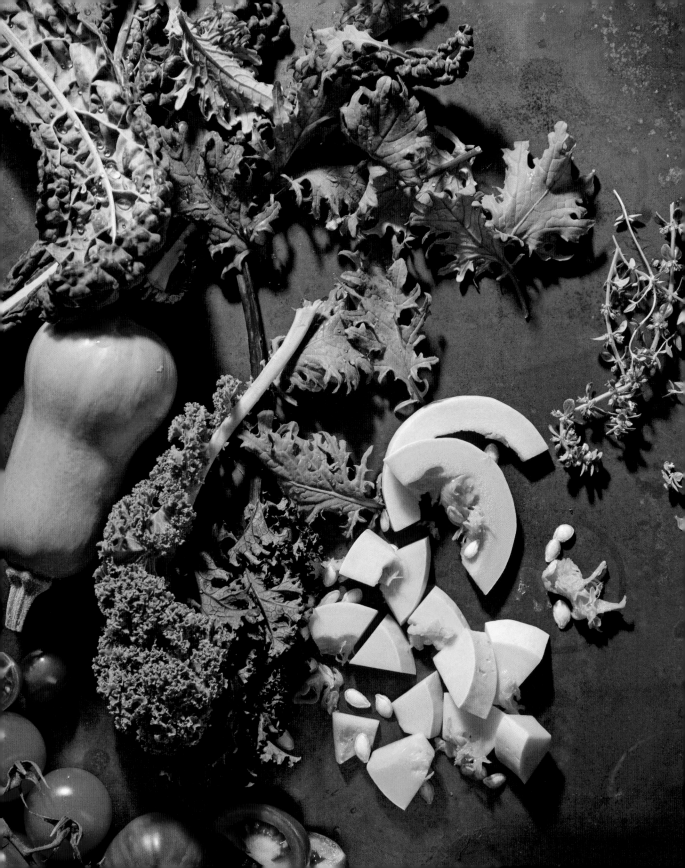

FALL RATATOUILLE

■ HEAL
■ WEIGHT LOSS
■ DETOX

2 tablespoons olive oil

1 onion, diced

1 clove garlic, minced

1 tablespoon tomato paste

½ teaspoon cumin seeds, crushed

1 tablespoon chopped fresh rosemary or ½ teaspoon dried

1 teaspoon sea salt

Ground black pepper, to taste

2 cups bite-size pieces butternut squash

2 cups water

4 tomatoes (about 3 cups chopped) or 1 can (14 ounces) diced or crushed tomatoes

2 cups thinly sliced curly or Lacinato kale (see "How to Prep Kale" for the best way to slice kale)

1. In a large pot over medium heat, warm the oil. Cook the onion, stirring, for 10 minutes, or until it is soft and translucent. Add the garlic and cook for 1 minute, or until fragrant. Stir in the tomato paste, cumin, rosemary, salt, and pepper and cook for 2 minutes, or until fragrant.

2. Stir in the butternut squash and cook, stirring frequently, for 15 minutes, or until the squash is tender. Add the water and tomatoes. Increase the heat to high and bring to a boil. Reduce the heat to low, add the kale, and simmer for 25 minutes, or until the mixture thickens and the squash is very soft and falling apart.

3. Enjoy warm or chilled.

This is my favorite escape in the fall when that back-to-school energy sets in and can become frenetic at times. Remind yourself that the relaxing days of summer aren't so far behind you and that fall brings lovely new gifts, as well. This savory soup combines late-season tomatoes and kale with a welcome new flavor that signals fall has arrived—hello, butternut squash!

HOW TO PREP KALE
Roll several kale leaves lengthwise. Using the point of your knife, cut away the thick center stem and discard it. Roll the remaining deveined leaves into tight little cigar shapes, and then slice into thin ribbons. This is the same technique as the chiffonade you tried with the Minty Melon Chia soup on page 132, with an extra step to remove the tough stem of the kale leaf here.

the freshness of your spices makes an unbelievable difference in adding depth of flavor to a rich stew like this. Buying spices in their whole form and then grinding or grating as needed for recipes is the best way to guarantee the freshest flavor. Buy whole nutmeg and cinnamon sticks, and grind them with a Microplane or the finest blade on a standard box grater. Look for whole cumin seeds in your grocery store, and use a coffee grinder or small food processor to grind them into a powder. Or hand-crush with a mortar and pestle.

MUSHROOM STEW
with STEEL-CUT OATS

2 tablespoons olive oil

1 yellow onion, chopped

1 clove garlic, chopped

2½ pounds mixed mushrooms (portobello, oyster, and shiitake are my favorite), roughly chopped

2 ribs celery, chopped

4 sprigs fresh rosemary, stems removed and leaves chopped

Pinch of red-pepper flakes

Pinch of ground black pepper

2 teaspoons sea salt

2 quarts water

⅓ cup steel-cut oats

Juice of ½ lemon

1. In a large pot over medium heat, warm the oil. Cook the onion and garlic, stirring frequently, for 5 to 7 minutes, or until the mixture is soft and translucent. Add the mushrooms, celery, rosemary, red-pepper flakes, black pepper, salt, and cook, stirring frequently, for 10 minutes, or until the celery is soft and the mushrooms are soft and browned. Stir in the water and cook for 5 minutes.

2. Using an immersion blender, puree the soup until slightly smooth. Or puree a quarter of the mixture in a countertop blender and then add back to the pot.

3. Stir in the oats and lemon juice, cover, and cook for 15 to 20 minutes, or until the oats are soft but still have a little bite. The oats will continue to soften and release starch even after the heat is turned off, and the soup will be rich and thick in texture and flavor.

I use mushrooms a lot. I do my best to shop organic, especially with mushrooms because they really absorb whatever is in the soil they sprout from. Organic means you won't be getting pesticides and other chemicals in your 'shrooms. Mushrooms are sui generis. There really isn't a vegetable out there that mimics the flavor and texture of a mushroom. If you don't like them, you could substitute kabocha squash or sweet potatoes plus spinach. I find the combination of a sweet and starchy squash or sweet potato along with the gentle bitterness of spinach creates an umami flavor similar to that of mushrooms. Umami—that "fifth taste" after sweet, sour, salty, and bitter—describes the unctuous flavor most often associated with meat, Parmigiano Reggiano, and even toasted nuts. Mushrooms have a trademark umami flavor, which is one of the reasons I gravitate toward them.

what exactly are steel-cut oats? They are chopped whole oat groats, and despite taking longer to cook, these oats have a superior nutty flavor to the regular rolled and quick oats. Steel-cut oats are less processed, and while they have the same amount of fiber and protein as the more processed rolled and quick oats, they do have more calcium.

Steel-cut oats can be used as a rice substitute to make risotto, pilaf, or other dishes that call for rice. You could even try them instead of the quinoa in the Mung and Quinoa Congee on page 91.

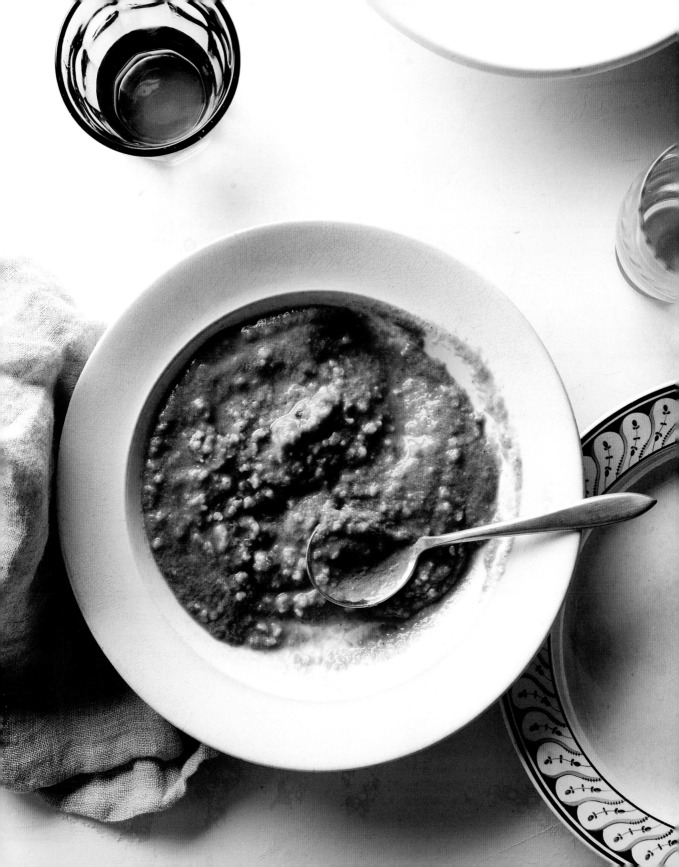

mindful movement

**Embracing challenges, and moving deeper into them,
will make you stronger while making the challenge easier.**

Our bodies want to resist change because of our biology; continuing to do something that is habit is a safer bet than trying something new and unproven. It's a way of protecting us from potential harm, but it also makes it tough to change even when we know better. Sometimes kicking up the intensity just a tad is all you need to push deeper into this broader challenge of improving your health. Start your soup ritual with five to 10 pushups or jumping jacks every day. You will get a quick rush of endorphins, and even though doing pushups and souping is a little harder than just souping, you just might find that it feels a little more fun.

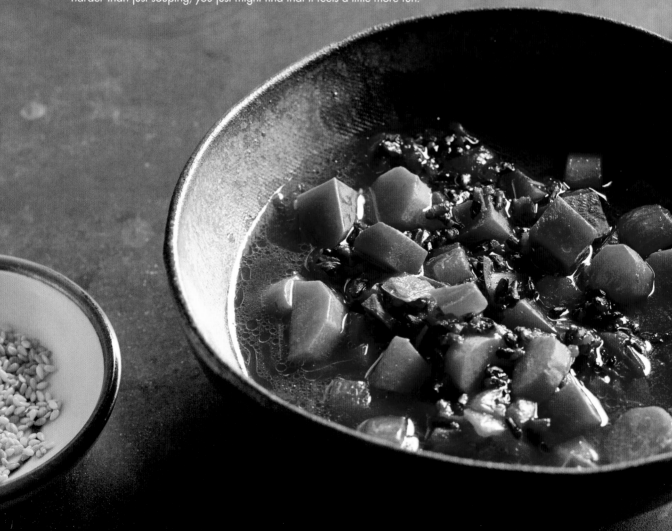

BLACK RICE WITH BEETS
and SESAME SEEDS

■ ENERGIZE
■ DETOX
■ MOM AND BABY

Beets shine like ruby-red jewels among the deep, black grains of rice, and little sprinkles of sesame seeds add in a toasty complement to the rich Middle Eastern spices.

2   tablespoons olive oil

2   leeks, white parts only, thinly sliced (about 1½ cups)

3   cloves garlic, minced

1   teaspoon sea salt

    Pinch of ground black pepper

2   tablespoons za'atar or 1 teaspoon dried oregano, 1 teaspoon dried thyme, 1 teaspoon sesame seeds, and 2 teaspoons sumac

1   carrot, diced

1   large beet, peeled and diced (about 3 cups)

¼   cup plus 1 quart water

2   tablespoons tahini

⅓   cup black rice or mixed wild rice, rinsed in a sieve until the water runs clear and soaked while preparing the other ingredients

    Peel of 1 lemon, grated (about 2 teaspoons)

1. In a large pot over medium heat, warm the oil. Cook the leeks and garlic, stirring occasionally, for 5 to 7 minutes, or until the mixture is soft and translucent. Stir in the salt, pepper, and za'atar and cook for 2 minutes, or until fragrant.

2. Stir in the carrot and beet and cook for 15 minutes, or until the vegetables are tender.

3. In a small bowl, add ¼ cup of the water and the tahini and stir to dissolve. Add to the pot and stir to combine.

4. Stir in the rice and the remaining quart water. Increase the heat to high and bring the water to a boil. Reduce the heat to low, cover, and simmer for 35 minutes, or until the rice is tender but still has some bite to it (al dente).

5. Serve warm with a sprinkle of the lemon peel.

sesame seeds are rich in vitamins, minerals, fat, protein, and carbohydrates, making them the perfect well-rounded seed to incorporate into your diet. While they're most known for decorating bagels and the tops of hamburger buns in American cuisine, sesame seeds and their oil are prominent in cuisines around the world, from the Middle East and Asia to the Caribbean and parts of Africa.

GREEN COCONUT CURRY
with **BROCCOLI**

Light sweetness from the coconut's rich milk and oil combine with green leafy flavors from broccoli and bok choy and fresh curry spices. The most beautiful curries are the ones made with freshly ground spices, but if you don't have time, you can find green Thai curry paste at an Asian grocer or order ahead online.

2 tablespoons coconut oil

1 large onion, diced

1 jalapeño pepper, seeded and finely chopped (use gloves if your skin is sensitive to hot peppers)

3 cloves garlic, minced

1 tablespoon grated fresh ginger

2 tablespoons green curry powder or paste

1 head broccoli, broken into small florets (about 4 cups)

¼ cup plus 1 quart water

1 can (15 ounces) coconut milk

Sea salt and ground black pepper, to taste

1 head bok choy, green leaves only, thinly sliced (about 4 cups)

¼ cup chopped fresh cilantro (optional)

1. In a large pot over medium heat, warm the oil. Cook the onion and pepper, stirring occasionally, for 5 to 7 minutes, or until the onion is soft and translucent. Add the garlic and ginger and cook, stirring, for 2 minutes, or until fragrant.

2. Stir in the green curry powder, broccoli, and ¼ cup of the water, cover, and cook for 5 minutes while occasionally stirring.

3. Add the coconut milk, salt, black pepper, and the remaining 1 quart water. Increase the heat to high and bring to a boil. Reduce the heat to medium to simmer. Add the bok choy and cover. Reduce the heat to low and cook for 15 minutes, or until the broccoli and bok choy are tender but still al dente.

4. Enjoy warm or chilled topped with the cilantro, if using. Add a few slices of fresh jalapeño pepper for more heat!

FRESH GREEN CURRY RECIPE

Green curry is native to Thailand, and you can buy it as a paste in a jar. Or you can make it from scratch. There's nothing like the taste and smell that comes from grinding these wet and dry aromatics together into a paste, plus you'll get a good forearm workout in the process. The flavor of green curry is more fresh than spicy, but you could add a jalapeño pepper to the mix to give it some heat. In a large mortar and pestle or on a large cutting board, add 1 tablespoon each cilantro stems, chopped garlic, chopped galangal (or ginger), and grated peel and juice of a kaffir lime (or a regular lime); 1 sliced shallot; ½ teaspoon each ground coriander and cumin; 1 teaspoon salt; and 5 or 6 green Thai chile peppers or 2 green bell peppers. Grind or chop into a paste. Oh, and you could also do this in a food processor; just add everything at once, and then pulse until combined.

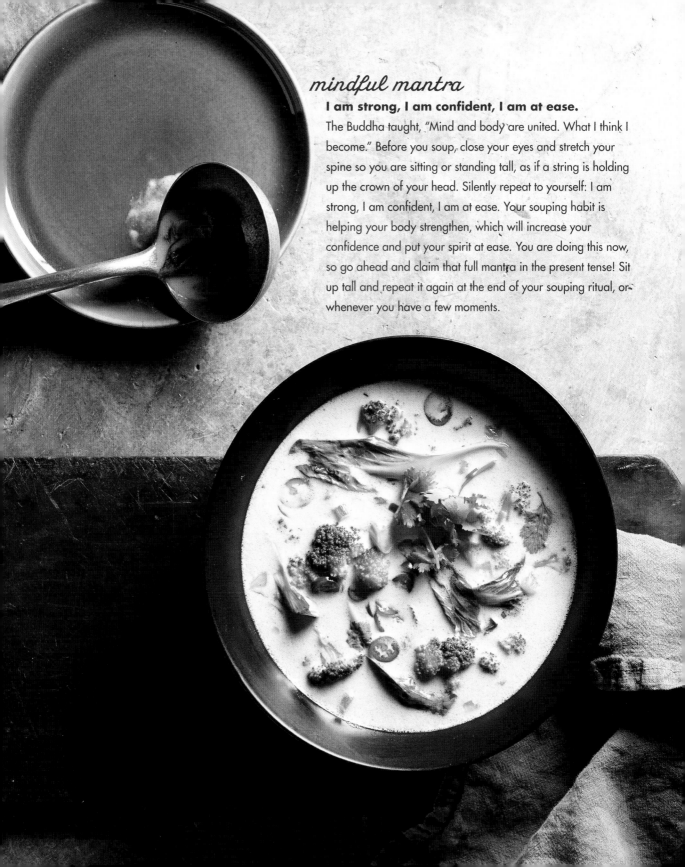

mindful mantra

I am strong, I am confident, I am at ease.
The Buddha taught, "Mind and body are united. What I think I become." Before you soup, close your eyes and stretch your spine so you are sitting or standing tall, as if a string is holding up the crown of your head. Silently repeat to yourself: I am strong, I am confident, I am at ease. Your souping habit is helping your body strengthen, which will increase your confidence and put your spirit at ease. You are doing this now, so go ahead and claim that full mantra in the present tense! Sit up tall and repeat it again at the end of your souping ritual, or whenever you have a few moments.

mindful mantra

As I engage with the unexpected, I reveal more of my potential.

Repeat this mantra as you make your cleanse menu, select ingredients, and prepare your soup. Repeat it as you soup. This mantra acknowledges each moment that you do something new and strengthens your connection to this newness. When you slow down to engage with each movement involved with the soup ritual you are forming, you might even find that time slows down. Enjoy this extra space and recognize it as an opening for you to move further on your journey to revealing your Splendid Self.

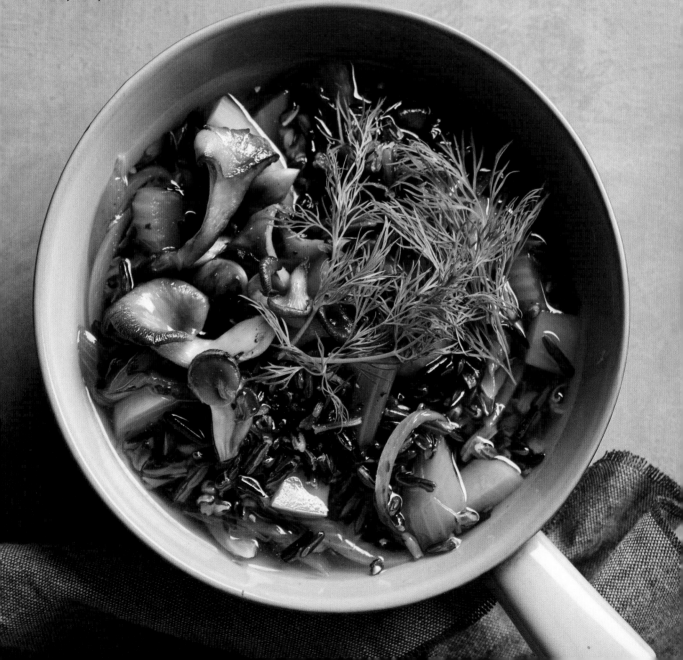

"CHICKEN" STEW
with RICE

2 tablespoons olive oil

1 yellow onion, diced

3 cloves garlic, minced

2 carrots, diced

2 large ribs celery, diced

1 teaspoon sea salt

½ teaspoon ground black pepper

1 teaspoon dried oregano

½ teaspoon dried thyme

3 cups king oyster mushrooms or regular oyster mushrooms or maitake mushrooms, chopped (about 10 ounces)

4 cups homemade vegetable stock or low-sodium store-bought broth

2 cups water

⅓ cup wild rice or short-grain brown rice, rinsed

¼ cup chopped fresh dill or 1 teaspoon dried

Lemon wedges (optional)

1. In a large pot over medium heat, warm the oil. Cook the onion, garlic, carrots, and celery, stirring frequently, for 7 to 10 minutes, or until the mixture is tender. Add the salt, pepper, oregano, and thyme and cook, stirring, for 2 minutes.

2. Add the mushrooms and cook for 10 minutes, or until the mushrooms have softened and browned a bit. This step is what really develops the flavor of your soup, so give it a little more time to make sure the mushrooms get color.

3. Stir in the stock and water. Increase the heat to high and bring to a boil. Reduce the heat to medium-low, stir in the rice, cover, and cook for 45 minutes, or until the rice is soft but still has some bite to it (al dente).

4. Stir in the dill at the last minute and serve warm with the lemon wedges, if using.

■ HEAL
■ WEIGHT LOSS
■ MOM AND BABY

Ask anyone what the best food is when feeling under the weather, and I guarantee the most common answer will be some variation of chicken soup. This soup focuses on the comfortable simplicity of chicken soup by highlighting the classic flavor combination of dill, celery, carrot, and onion and increasing the nutrient density with wild rice (or short-grain brown rice if you like your rice to fall apart a bit more in your soup). And, of course, the chicken replacement: king oyster mushrooms. King oyster mushrooms are tall, cylindrical mushrooms that bear an uncanny resemblance to chicken in this soup. They have a light-colored flesh that is a little more dense than some other mushrooms, and they soak up the flavors of the broth and seasonings beautifully. That's a big part of why we like chicken: It doesn't have a terribly strong flavor, but it acts as a nice, chewy vehicle to get more of that soup flavor onto our taste buds. Regular oyster mushrooms work well here, too, as do maitake (also known as "hen of the woods") mushrooms.

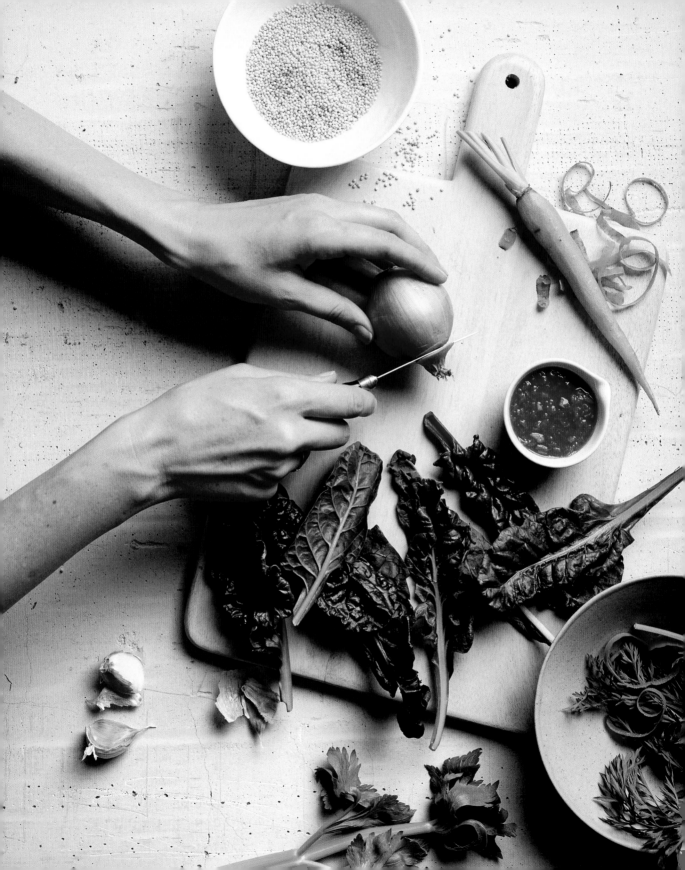

RAINBOW CHARD STEW
with HARISSA-INFUSED MILLET

There is something a little enchanting about seeing bunches of rainbow chard heaped together in piles at the market. If you haven't seen rainbow chard in person, the name gives a clue to its allure; the stems sprout in vibrant shades of pink, yellow, white, and purple. The Technicolor piles are a field day for foodie photographers. Swiss chard is the same as rainbow chard, so you don't need all the beautiful color to get your cleanse on. Chard is a hardy leafy green that can withstand both really warm and really cool temperatures, so its growing season is long in most climates.

2 tablespoons olive oil

1 yellow onion, diced

2 large ribs celery, diced

3 cloves garlic, minced

2 tablespoons harissa pepper sauce or 1 teaspoon red-pepper flakes, 1 teaspoon caraway seeds, and ½ teaspoon ground coriander

1 bunch rainbow chard, tough stems removed and roughly chopped into bite-size pieces (about 5 cups)

1 teaspoon sea salt

Ground black pepper, to taste

4 cups Vegan Bone Broth (page 174) or low-sodium store-bought broth

2 cups water

⅓ cup millet

1. In a large pot over medium heat, warm the oil. Cook the onion and celery, stirring frequently, for 5 to 7 minutes, or until the mixture is soft and translucent. Stir in the garlic and harissa and cook for 1 to 2 minutes, or until fragrant.

2. Add the chard, salt, and pepper and cook, stirring frequently, for 10 minutes, or until the chard leaves are wilted and the stems are soft.

3. Stir in the broth and water. Increase the heat to high and bring to a boil. Reduce the heat to medium-low, add the millet, cover, and cook for 25 minutes, or until the millet is soft.

4. Serve warm.

harissa is hands down my favorite spicy condiment. It's a little like curry in that the primary ingredients are often the same, but it can be blended in countless ways, with or without some add-ins. It is a staple in Tunisian cuisine and typically includes a blend of spicy and smoked chile peppers, garlic, olive oil, cumin, caraway seeds, and coriander. It can also contain mint, tomatoes, and rose petals. My favorite jar of the moment is a blend from the brand Mina.

CRANBERRY BEANS *and* KABOCHA SQUASH STEW

4 cups chopped kabocha squash or pumpkin or butternut squash

3 tablespoons olive oil, divided

1 small yellow onion, diced

3 cloves garlic, minced

1 tablespoon finely chopped fresh sage

1 teaspoon ground cinnamon

½ teaspoon red-pepper flakes (more if you like heat)

1 cup fresh cranberry beans or soaked dried cranberry beans (they must be soaked overnight, rinsed, and drained) or 1 can (15 ounces) low-sodium chickpeas or cannellini beans, rinsed and drained

1 quart water (add 2 cups if using dried beans)

1 teaspoon sea salt (omit if using canned beans)

1. Preheat the oven to 400°F.

2. On a baking sheet, toss the squash or pumpkin with 1 tablespoon of the oil and spread into a single layer. Cook for 40 minutes, stirring halfway through, or until the squash or pumpkin is tender when pierced with a fork. Set aside to cool.

3. While the squash is cooking, in a medium pot over medium heat, warm the remaining 2 tablespoons oil. Cook the onion, stirring, for 5 to 7 minutes, or until it is tender and translucent. Add the garlic, sage, cinnamon, and red-pepper flakes and stir for 1 minute, or until fragrant.

4. Add the beans and stir to combine. (You can use canned beans here and continue the recipe as is, but if you use dried beans, you will need to add 2 cups of the water at this point and cook for 45 minutes before adding the squash or pumpkin.)

5. Add the water and reserved squash or pumpkin. Increase the heat to high and bring to a boil. Reduce the heat to medium and simmer for 45 minutes, or until the stew has thickened and the beans are tender. Stir in the salt.

6. Serve hot.

■ STRENGTHEN
■ MOM AND BABY

Fresh beans are fun to work with because they don't need as much prep time as dried beans, which have been taken from their shells and dried to extend their life span. That never-been-dried flavor is very different than what you might be used to with dried or canned beans—and in all the ways you might expect. The texture is springier and more tender, while the flavor is a cleaner and clearer vegetal note and less starchy. The fresh cranberry beans play nicely with the grown-up flavor of the kabocha squash. Kabocha is a hard squash available the same time of year as butternut squash and pumpkins. It has a darker, more pebbly skin than almost any other squash you might see at the market. If you are intimidated by the thought of peeling it, cut it in half, scoop the seeds out, rub it with olive oil, and roast it (covered with foil) for about 1 hour. Then just spoon out the soft flesh to use in this recipe.

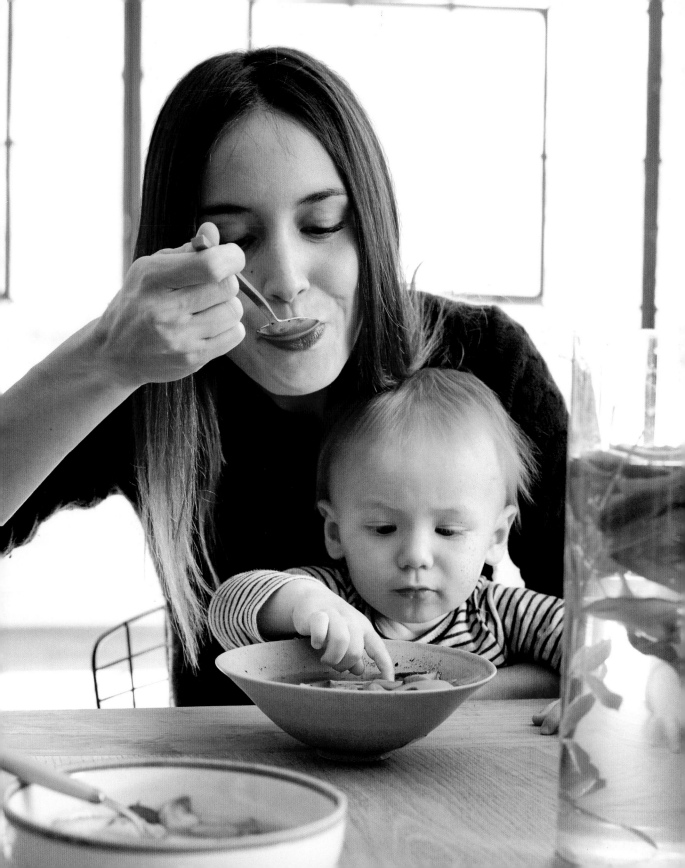

POTATO *and* CABBAGE PAPRIKASH

This recipe is inspired by a Hungarian dish that is traditionally full of cream and chicken. It's delicious and puts me to sleep every time I eat it. Amazingly, this soup is also super creamy while managing to be incredibly energizing. Everything in this soup from the cashew cream to the cabbage to the potatoes will stick to your ribs without clinging to your waist, if you know what I mean. It's magic.

- 2   tablespoons olive oil
- 1   onion, diced
- 3   cloves garlic, minced
- 1   teaspoon sea salt
- ¼   teaspoon caraway seeds, crushed
- 1   teaspoon sweet Hungarian paprika (see note)
     Ground black pepper, to taste
- 2   cups shredded green cabbage
- 2   cups oyster mushrooms, chopped into bite-size pieces (about 4 ounces)
- 1   cup chopped new potatoes
- 1   quart plus 1 cup water
- ½   cup cashews, soaked overnight and drained (see "Why Soak Your Nuts and Seeds?" on page 74 for more information)
- 1   tablespoon apple cider vinegar
- ¼   cup chopped fresh flat-leaf parsley (optional)

1. In a large pot over medium heat, warm the oil. Cook the onion and garlic for 5 to 7 minutes, or until the mixture is soft and fragrant.

2. Add the salt, caraway seeds, paprika, and pepper and stir for 1 minute. Add the cabbage and cook for 10 to 15 minutes, or until the cabbage is wilted. Add the mushrooms and cook for 6 minutes, or until the mushrooms are soft.

3. Stir in the potatoes and 1 quart of the water. Increase the heat to high and bring to a boil. Reduce the heat to medium and simmer for 25 minutes, or until the potatoes are falling apart and the cabbage is very soft.

4. In a countertop blender, combine the cashews with the remaining 1 cup water and puree until smooth. Stir the cashew cream and apple cider vinegar into the pot off the heat.

5. Sprinkle with the parsley, if using, and serve warm.

Note: Sweet paprika (like the Hungarian variety called for in this recipe) is the most common, and it is a mix of dried peppers that have been ground into a fine powder. There's also smoked paprika (also called pimenton, from Spain), which uses smoked peppers to yield that characteristic heady flavor and aroma you taste in paella, and spicy paprika, which is just sweet paprika that includes ground red pepper. All paprikas contain a mix of different peppers and in varying proportions, so try a few and pick the one that suits your taste buds best.

mindful moment

We can always come back to our breath. The leaves fade, the days shorten, and the air cools, but the trees are still there, rooted in the same ground that was hot in the summer and frosty on a fall morning. Our breath is a reminder that we are trees, too; our environment around us is dynamic, but we are here, breathing, capable of accepting the unexpected as simply a part of our existence. Before and after your soup meal, set the timer for 5 minutes and focus on your breath. Breathe in, pause, exhale out, pause, breathe in. You will find a pace, and the purpose is to simply guide your thoughts back to your breath whenever your mind wanders. Your breath is a constant, gentle reminder that you can be still and rooted regardless of the dynamic environment around you.

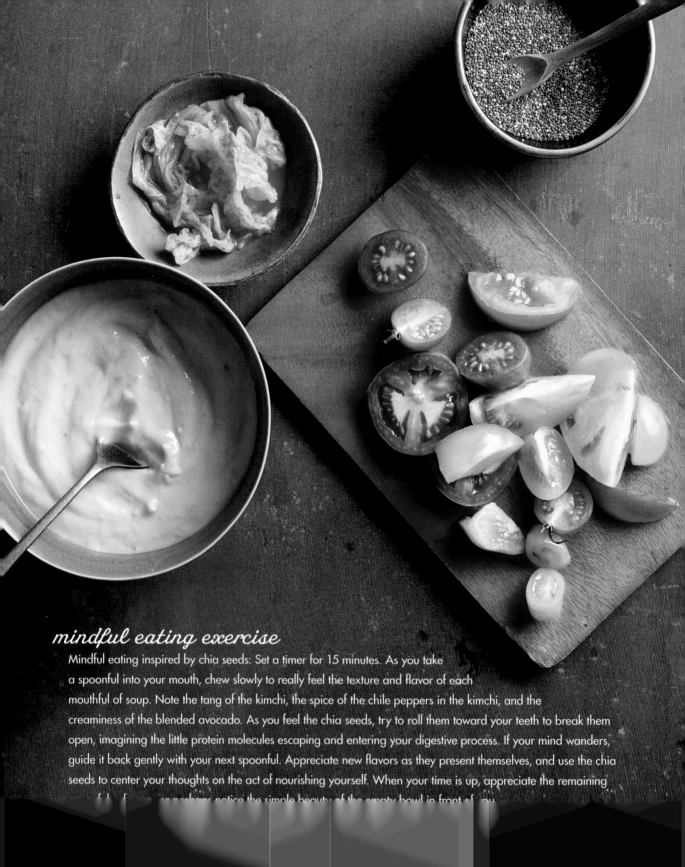

mindful eating exercise

Mindful eating inspired by chia seeds: Set a timer for 15 minutes. As you take
a spoonful into your mouth, chew slowly to really feel the texture and flavor of each
mouthful of soup. Note the tang of the kimchi, the spice of the chile peppers in the kimchi, and the
creaminess of the blended avocado. As you feel the chia seeds, try to roll them toward your teeth to break them
open, imagining the little protein molecules escaping and entering your digestive process. If your mind wanders,
guide it back gently with your next spoonful. Appreciate new flavors as they present themselves, and use the chia
seeds to center your thoughts on the act of nourishing yourself. When your time is up, appreciate the remaining

AVOCADO KIMCHI STEW

4   very ripe avocados, halved and flesh scooped out

2   scallions, roughly chopped

Juice of 2 limes

2½ cups water

Sea salt and ground black pepper, to taste

3   tomatoes, diced (save as much juice as possible; seeds are fine), about 3½ cups

1   cup kimchi

1   tablespoon chia seeds

1. In a countertop blender, combine the avocados, scallions, lime juice, and water and puree until very smooth. Season with the salt and pepper. Stir in the tomatoes.

2. Put ¼ cup of the kimchi in a bowl and pour the avocado soup around it. Sprinkle with the chia seeds.

As this is one of my few raw recipes, I recommend enjoying this soup within 3 days of making it since nutrient loss in cut raw vegetables is much more rapid than with cooked. Its creamy, savory texture is the perfect counterpoint to the spicy, tangy, crunchy kimchi. If you have never tried kimchi, use this as your chance. You can find it in the refrigerated aisle of many large grocery stores now, and there is usually a vegan variety. (Traditionally, kimchi is made with oysters.) Kimchi represents one of the oldest forms of food preservation in which the vegetable (cabbage in this case) ferments with the help of the bacteria that proliferate as it decomposes. Just like yogurt, kimchi is an amazing source of probiotics—the healthy bacteria that you want to promote growth of in your belly.

CHIA SEEDS AS A GARNISH

I like whole chia seeds as a garnish for this stew for their crunchy texture, but you will need to chew more slowly and intentionally if you want to break through those little seed shells to get at the nutrients locked inside the seeds. (Remember, chia seeds and flaxseeds are usually ground before adding to any recipe for this reason.) You could use this as a mindful eating exercise! If you choose to stir the chia seeds into your blended soup instead of sprinkling them as a crunchy topper, that's okay, too. They will slowly become gelatinous and create a more porridgelike consistency.

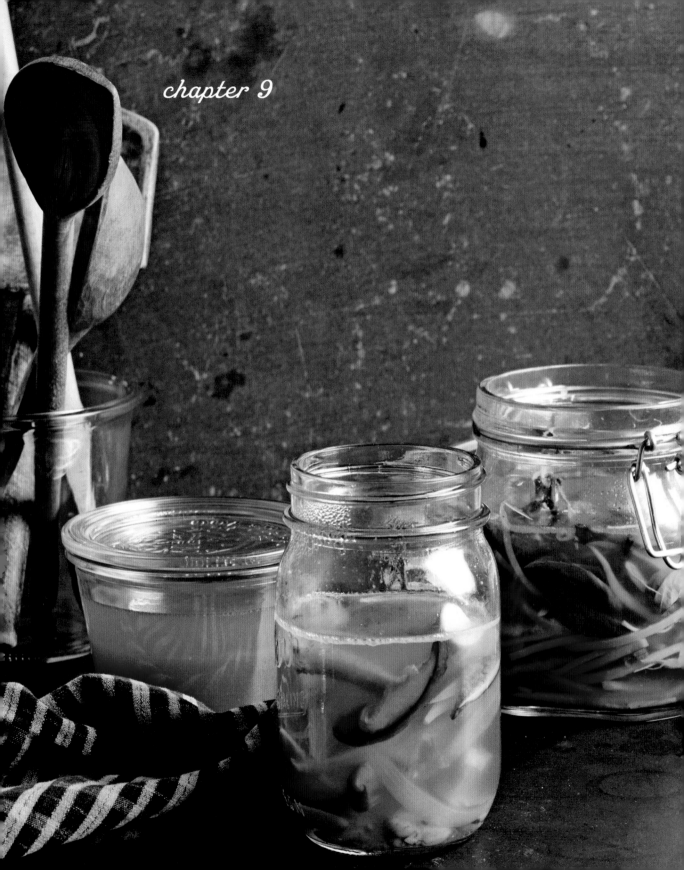

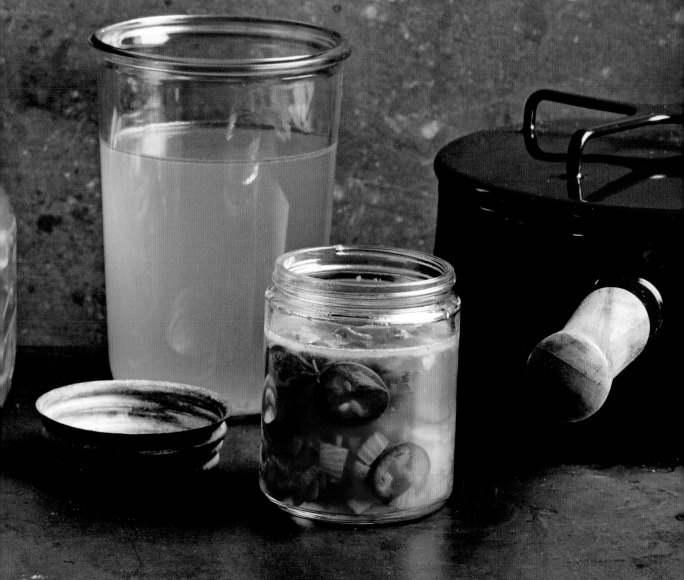

chapter 9

RESTORATIVE BROTHS

broths have a few different names depending on where you are spooning: dashi, stock, bouillon. They all mean water plus a variety of vegetables and herbs (and often meat) cooked at a gentle simmer for a period of time to draw flavor from the ingredients. Of course, at Splendid Spoon we don't add meat because we're really focused on simple plant-based nutrition (and simply adding more veggies to your diet!), but the process and goals are very similar. Broths are like an elixir in this way: They appear watery and clear, but they carry a variety of flavors. I find broths to be a bit like teas in their effect. They are calming, and they feel like more of a ritual. For this reason, we really love closing a day of souping with broth at Splendid Spoon. Pour it into a mug steaming hot, and first appreciate the aromas lifting out and around you. That first deep breath of herbs and vegetables and warmth is very soothing. You might pick a broth with more ginger if you are fending off a cold or tend to crave a spicier flavor at the end of the day. Or perhaps a broth with more vegetables is what you crave so you end your day with the satisfying crunch of carrots or radishes.

Broths are lighter in consistency and flavor than my other soups, but I rarely strain out the vegetables so you get more fiber and lots of interesting textures to chew on. I don't include much salt in these broths to create a truly hydrating experience as you sip before bedtime. You can keep a little dish of sea salt, or even smoked salt, at the ready for a touch more salinity as you sip or spoon your broth. I'll never go to bed with a grumbling tummy. Ending the day with a belly full of warm broth helps me relax into a peaceful state of rest.

These broths can also be used instead of water in any of the recipes in this book. They will add more dimension and flavor, and I suggest omitting the salt in your broth recipe if you plan to use it in the cooking process for another soup. I call for the Vegan Bone Broth (page 174) in some of the other recipes in this book because its flavor is mild and complementary to many recipes, but feel free to use whichever broth you like best!

DAIKON RADISH WITH TAMARIND *and* SPINACH

Crisp and tangy with a peppery kick, this soup has a light and fresh feel. Tart tamarind plays with slightly floral grated lime peel, and daikon bites back with a peppery kick that is typical of most vegetables in the radish family. I use a lot of cilantro as garnish to accentuate the green flavor of the spinach, but you could also use parsley or mint, or a combination of the three.

2	tablespoons sesame oil or olive oil
4	scallions, thinly sliced
1	clove garlic, minced
3	cups diced daikon radish or red radish
½	teaspoon red-pepper flakes
½	teaspoon sea salt
½	teaspoon tamarind paste
2	quarts water
4	cups loosely packed baby spinach
1	teaspoon grated lime peel
1	cup chopped fresh cilantro

1. In a large pot over medium heat, warm the oil. Cook the scallions and garlic for 1 minute, or until fragrant.

2. Stir in the radish, red-pepper flakes, and salt. Reduce the heat to low and cook for 10 minutes, or until the radish is soft.

3. Add the tamarind paste and stir to combine. Stir in the water to dissolve the paste. Increase the heat to high and bring to a boil. Reduce the heat to medium-low and simmer for 10 minutes.

4. Stir in the spinach and lime peel, turn off the heat, and cover for 5 minutes before serving.

5. Top with a generous sprinkle of the cilantro.

daikon radishes are high in enzymes that aid in the digestion of fat and starch. They contain high amounts of vitamin C, potassium, and phosphorus and have been shown to aid in the relief of migraines by opening up constricted blood vessels.

tamarind also contains tartaric acid, just as citrus fruits contain citric acid, providing not just a zing to the taste buds but also powerful antioxidant action, zapping harmful free radicals floating through your system.

VEGAN BONE BROTH

2–3 ounces dried mushrooms (any variety)

5 cups boiled water

2 tablespoons olive oil

1 large onion, diced, or 1 cup onion ends

2 carrots, diced, or 2 cups carrot ends

2 ribs celery, diced, or 2 cups celery ends

4 cups shiitake mushrooms, sliced

3 cloves garlic, smashed

3 tablespoons grated fresh ginger

1 teaspoon ground cumin

1 teaspoon dried rosemary

3 cups spinach, chopped

3 cups chopped bok choy

1 cup loosely packed Thai basil leaves or Italian basil

Pinch of sea salt

2½ quarts water

Juice of ½ lemon

½ teaspoon spirulina powder (see note)

1. In a small bowl, soak the dried mushrooms in the boiled water for 15 minutes, or until they are soft. Remove the mushrooms and reserve the water. Slice the mushrooms.

2. In a large pot over medium heat, warm the oil. Cook the onion, carrots, and celery, stirring, for 5 to 7 minutes, or until the mixture is tender.

3. Add the shiitake mushrooms, garlic, ginger, cumin, and rosemary and cook, stirring, for 5 minutes, or until fragrant.

4. Add the soaked mushrooms and soaking water, spinach, bok choy, basil, salt, and water. Increase the heat to high and bring to a boil. Reduce the heat to low and simmer for 1 hour, or until the broth is slightly thick and brownish green in color.

5. Turn off the heat, strain the liquid, and stir in the lemon juice and spirulina.

6. Sip slowly or use as a base for other soups.

Traditional bone broth uses animal bones that provide collagen and is purported to improve the health of the stomach and immune system. Actually, our bodies have to break down that collagen into amino acids before putting them to use where needed, and you can get all the same amino acids that make up collagen from plant sources. In addition to amino acid–rich greens and flavorful shiitakes, this vegan version includes onions and garlic, which contain prebiotic compounds to keep the microenvironment of your gut in balance. This recipe is a stock of sorts, so you can use vegetable "ends." When I call for an *end*, it simply means the tougher ends of the vegetable that you typically discard or throw into the compost heap. These bits of roughage will infuse your broth with both nutrients and flavor, plus using them reduces food waste!

Note: Spirulina is an antioxidant- and calcium-dense algae sold in powder form at most health food stores. For more on spirulina, see the "Plant Power" section in Chapter 2, page 31.

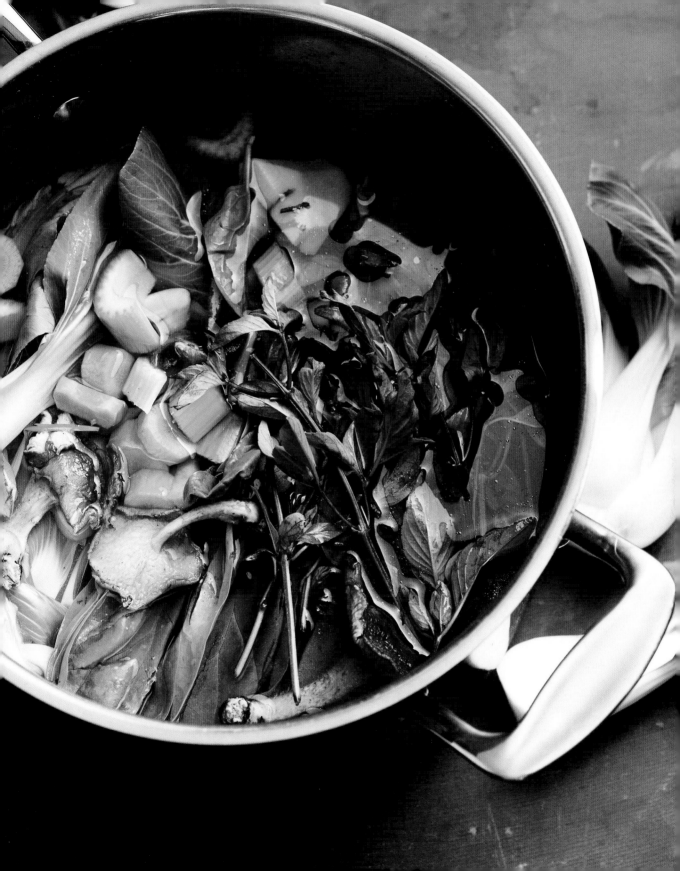

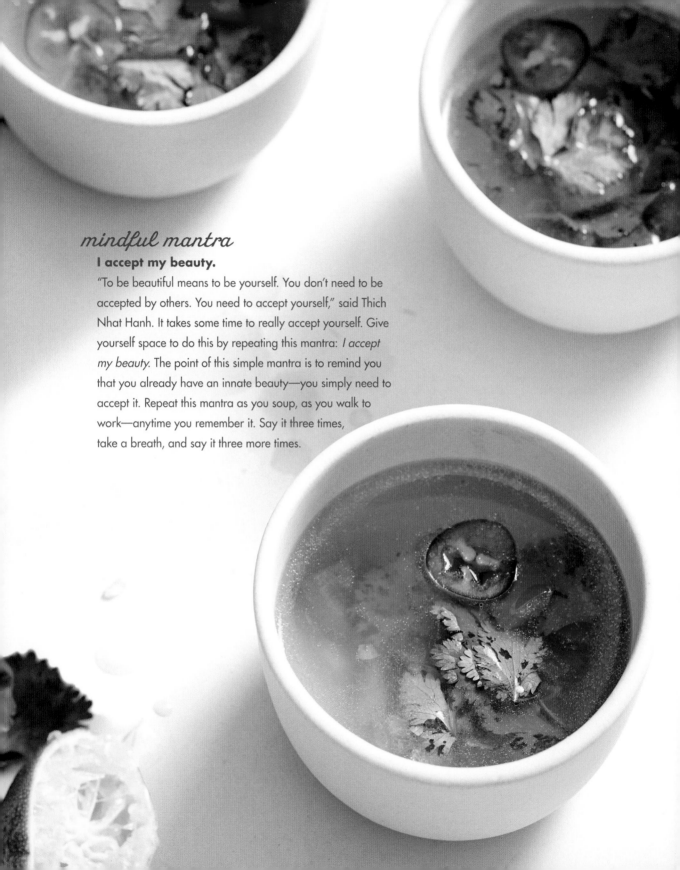

mindful mantra

I accept my beauty.

"To be beautiful means to be yourself. You don't need to be
accepted by others. You need to accept yourself," said Thich
Nhat Hanh. It takes some time to really accept yourself. Give
yourself space to do this by repeating this mantra: *I accept
my beauty.* The point of this simple mantra is to remind you
that you already have an innate beauty—you simply need to
accept it. Repeat this mantra as you soup, as you walk to
work—anytime you remember it. Say it three times,
take a breath, and say it three more times.

LIME PEPPER

1   tablespoon olive oil

1   onion, sliced

1   red bell pepper, diced into ½" pieces

2   cloves garlic, minced

1   tablespoon tomato paste

1   large tomato, diced

1   jalapeño pepper, seeded and finely chopped (use more or less depending on your penchant for spice, and keep the seeds in if you like to amp up the heat; use gloves if your skin is sensitive to hot peppers)

½   cup chopped fresh cilantro

1   teaspoon ground cumin

1   teaspoon sea salt

    Ground black pepper, to taste

2   quarts water

    Juice of 3 limes

Ohhh, this broth will just shake the cold right out of you. Mexican tortilla soup was the inspiration here, and who knew a humble broth could produce such tantalizing flavors? The zesty burst of lime, spicy little kick of jalapeño, and the freshness of cilantro work together to soothe your soul and revive your senses.

1. In a large pot over medium heat, warm the oil. Cook the onion, bell pepper, and garlic for 7 to 10 minutes, or until the mixture is soft. Add the tomato paste, tomato, and jalapeño pepper and cook, stirring, for 5 minutes, or until the peppers are soft.

2. Add the cilantro, cumin, salt, black pepper, and water. Increase the heat to high and bring to a boil. Reduce the heat to low and simmer for 10 minutes.

3. Turn off the heat and stir in the lime juice.

4. Enjoy warm or chilled.

adding some spicy chile peppers to a healthy meal may help you burn a few extra calories and a bit more fat. It isn't a magic bullet, but this modest boost in metabolism translates to about 100 extra burned calories a day for a 110-pound woman and 200 calories for a 200-pound man.

WAKAME BROTH *with* MUSHROOMS AND GREEN GARLIC

This vibrant broth is fresh like a spring morning thanks to the youthful bite of green garlic and wakame's sea-breeziness. Waka-*what*, you ask? Cultivated in Japan since the 8th century, this edible brown seaweed is a staple in Japanese, Korean, and Chinese cuisines and is loaded with magnesium, iodine, calcium, iron, and folate. Wakame imparts earthy, green flavors and vital minerals to this broth, complementing the grounding flavors of enoki and shiitake mushrooms.

1   tablespoon coconut oil

1   onion, sliced

2   stalks green garlic or scallions, thinly sliced

1   cup shiitake mushrooms, stems removed and caps thinly sliced

1   cup enoki mushrooms, roots removed and long stems separated (see note)

1   teaspoon sea salt

    Peel of 1 lime, grated (about 2 teaspoons)

    Red-pepper flakes, to taste

¼   cup dried wakame

2   quarts water

½   cup dried porcini mushrooms

    Juice of 1 lime

1. In a large pot over medium heat, warm the oil. Cook the onion and green garlic or scallions, stirring, for 5 to 7 minutes, or until the mixture is soft. Add the shiitake and enoki mushrooms and cook for 5 to 10 minutes, stirring halfway, or until the mushrooms are soft.

2. Add the salt, lime peel, red-pepper flakes, wakame, water, and dried mushrooms. Increase the heat to high and bring to a boil. Reduce the heat to low and simmer for 45 minutes.

3. Finish with the lime juice and enjoy warm!

Note: Don't bother chopping the enoki mushrooms; they are super delicate and will cook quickly while adding beautiful texture and visual interest to your soup.

CABBAGE BORSCHT

■ WEIGHT LOSS
■ DETOX

2 tablespoons olive oil

1 red onion, sliced

1 beet, shredded or thinly sliced (about 2 cups)

3 cups sliced red cabbage (about ⅓ head)

1 large carrot, shredded or julienned

¼ teaspoon dried thyme

½ teaspoon sea salt

   Pinch of ground black pepper

1 recipe Vegan Bone Broth (page 174) or 2 quarts low-sodium store-bought vegetable broth

¼ cup cashews, soaked overnight and drained (see "Why Soak Your Nuts and Seeds?" on page 74 for more information)

¾ cup water

1 tablespoon red wine vinegar

¼ cup chopped fresh dill

Aah, a good borscht on a rainy day will soothe you all the way down to your core. This iconic cabbage soup is of Ukrainian origin, and it is a staple in many Eastern and Central European cuisines. Cabbage dominates the rich flavor of this soup, but in most traditional recipes, it is made with beetroot as the main ingredient. Some regions feature tomato as the star, while beetroot plays second fiddle. Some varieties don't even use any beetroot at all, such as green borscht and white borscht.

1. In a large pot over medium heat, warm the oil. Cook the onion, beet, cabbage, carrot, thyme, salt, and pepper, stirring occasionally, for 12 to 15 minutes, or until the cabbage is soft.

2. Add the broth. Increase the heat to high and bring to a boil. Reduce the heat to medium and simmer for 1 hour, or until the vegetables are tender.

3. In a countertop blender or food processor, puree the cashews and water until very smooth.

4. Stir the vinegar and dill into the borscht. Top with the cashew cream and enjoy hot.

HOW TO SLICE CABBAGE

Cut off the hard end and peel away the outer layer of cabbage leaves. Slice the cabbage into three sections. Slice out the core at the center of each section and discard or throw it in your compost heap. Cut one section (or 3 cups' worth) into fine slices. (You can also use the large shredding attachment on your food processor or the large holes on your box grater.) Wrap the remaining two sections of cabbage in plastic wrap and store in the fridge. Or slice, steam, and freeze to lock in the nutrients and save for another borscht day.

CONFETTI PHO

1 recipe Vegan Bone Broth (page 174) or 2 quarts low-sodium store-bought vegetable broth

1 stalk lemongrass, smashed

1 tablespoon grated fresh ginger

1 cup spiralized or julienned or peeled carrot

1 cup spiralized or julienned or peeled turnip

½ cup sliced shiitake caps

1 scallion, sliced

Add to taste at the table:

Torn Thai basil leaves

Bean sprouts

Lime wedges

Sliced jalapeño pepper (use gloves if your skin is sensitive to hot peppers)

Mint leaves

1. In a large pot over high heat, bring the broth to a boil. Add the lemongrass, ginger, carrot, turnip, mushrooms, and scallion. Reduce the heat to low and simmer for 30 minutes, or until the mushrooms are soft and the veggie "noodles" are al dente.

2. Serve steaming hot in large bowls (make sure to pick bowls big enough to accommodate all the add-ons!) with toppings to your taste.

MAKING VEGETABLE NOODLES

Think you need a spiralizer here? Sure it will work, but there are other tricks to getting long, delicate vegetable "noodles."

- Use a julienne peeler.

- Go for matchstick-size pieces with your knife. Remember what I said in Chapter 4 about your cells not knowing the difference between a julienne and a chiffonade? There, I said it again. Thin-ish is just fine for this recipe.

- With a peeler, make pappardelle-style veggie ribbons that have a light noodle feel. These wider, thinner veggie noodles may be the easiest and prettiest of all!

WEIGHT LOSS
DETOX

There's a neighborhood near the town I grew up in named "the X" because of the crisscrossing intersections that can make it difficult to navigate. After you weave yourself through the X, there is a Vietnamese restaurant called Pho Saigon. On my first visit, as a total Vietnamese neophyte, I ordered the restaurant's eponymous dish. And an enormous bowl of scalding hot broth was set before me. Around it went huge leaves of basil, crisp sprout shoots, bright lime wedges, chile peppers, and, of course, a pile of noodles. The aroma of torn leaves and chile peppers and tart lime juice hitting that hot broth will make me giddy even on a day when I'm stuffed with a cold—and this is exactly the soup you will crave when your sinuses are throbbing. I look to replicate that first steamy encounter with every bowl I've had since. This version replaces the traditional rice noodles with a rainbow of root vegetables to up your plant quotient.

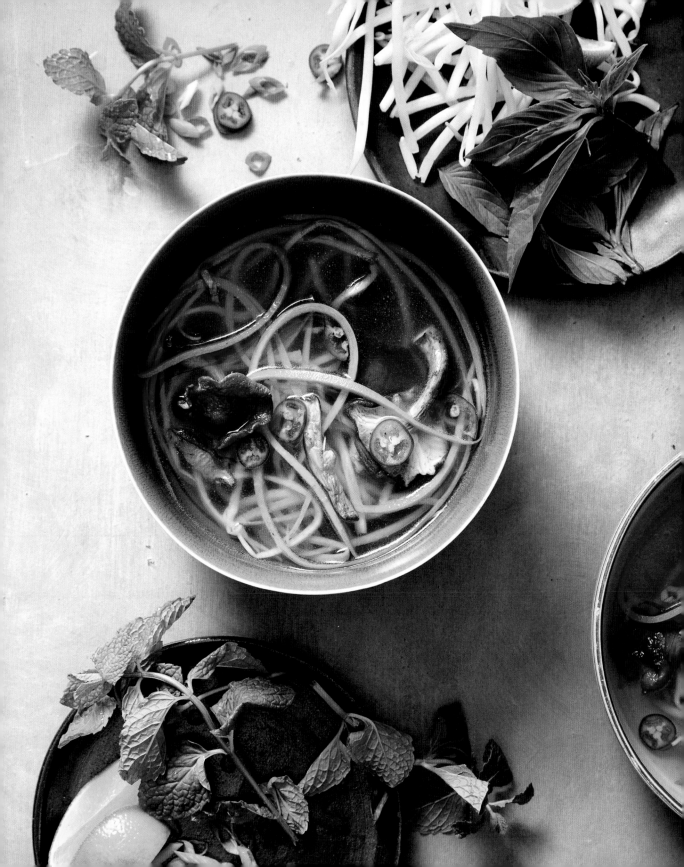

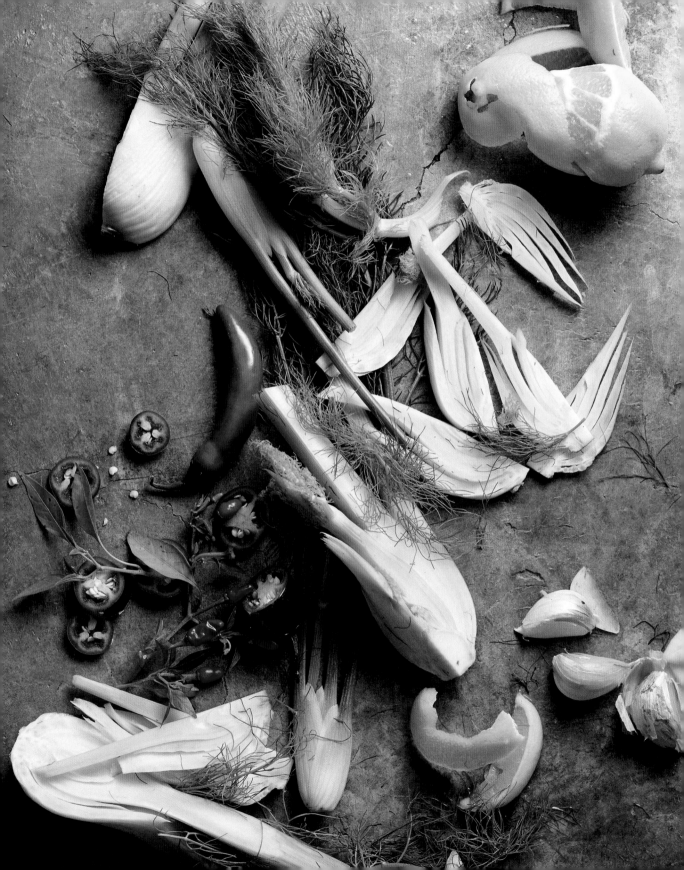

LEMON-FENNEL CONSOMMÉ

■ HEAL
■ WEIGHT LOSS
■ DETOX

This broth tastes like pure sunshine, with fresh citrus to awaken your senses and the toasty warmth of fennel.

2 tablespoons olive oil

1 yellow onion, sliced

1 clove garlic, smashed and chopped

1 fennel bulb, thinly sliced (a round one if you can find it; makes about 2½ cups)

2 quarts water

1 teaspoon sea salt

1 red chile pepper, any variety (use gloves if your skin is sensitive to hot peppers) or ½ teaspoon red-pepper flakes

Grated peel of 1 lemon

Grated peel and juice of 1 large orange

¼ cup chopped fresh dill

1. In a large pot over medium heat, warm the oil. Cook the onion, garlic, and fennel, stirring, for 5 to 7 minutes, or until the mixture is soft.

2. Add the water, salt, pepper, lemon peel, orange peel, and orange juice. Increase the heat to high and bring to a boil. Reduce the heat to low and simmer for 1 hour.

3. Stir in the dill and enjoy hot.

a traditional consommé is a type of clear soup made from richly flavored stock or bouillon that has been clarified, a process which uses egg whites to remove fat and sediment. Because this recipe is plant-based, the only fat comes from olive oil, and I leave the vegetable matter in there for texture and the nutritional benefits of dietary fiber. But you can definitely strain this soup for a really clear broth that looks like a traditional consommé. This will make it easier to use as a base broth in other recipes, as well.

PUMPKIN AND MUSHROOMS *with* STAR ANISE BROTH

■ **ENERGIZE**
■ **STRENGTHEN**
■ **MOM AND BABY**

Hello, autumn! Savor the changing seasons with every spoonful of this sweetly spiced broth. Pumpkin and butternut squash impart golden flavors rich with nostalgia and phytonutrients, while mushrooms add an earthy, meaty depth. Few other whole plants can compete with these hearty fungi.

2 tablespoons olive oil

1 small yellow onion, diced

1 clove garlic, minced

1 sprig rosemary, stems removed and finely chopped, or large pinch of dried rosemary

2 cups cubed (½") pumpkin or kabocha squash or butternut squash

2 large portobello mushroom caps, cut into bite-size pieces (about 3 cups)

1 teaspoon sea salt

2 quarts water

1 teaspoon ground cinnamon

Pinch of ground red pepper

2 full pods or stars of star anise (not just the seeds)

1 tablespoon grated fresh ginger

1. In a large pot over medium heat, warm the oil. Cook the onion and garlic, stirring, for 5 to 7 minutes, or until the mixture is very soft. Add the rosemary and cook for 1 minute, or until fragrant.

2. Add the pumpkin or squash, mushrooms, and salt and cook, stirring occasionally, for about 15 minutes, or until the mushrooms are soft.

3. Add the water, cinnamon, pepper, star anise, and ginger. Increase the heat to high and bring to a boil. Reduce the heat to medium-low and simmer for 1 hour, or until the pumpkin or squash is tender.

4. Remove the star anise pods, if you wish (I like to leave them in, but the pods themselves are not edible). Serve in warm bowls.

ginger is a good source of vitamin C, magnesium, potassium, copper, and manganese, and is listed as an herbal medicine with carminative effects, meaning it promotes the release of intestinal gas. It's also an intestinal spasmolytic, which relaxes and soothes the intestinal tract. That means it can settle an upset stomach, relieve vomiting, and ease gas and diarrhea. It's also effective in preventing nausea in the first place.

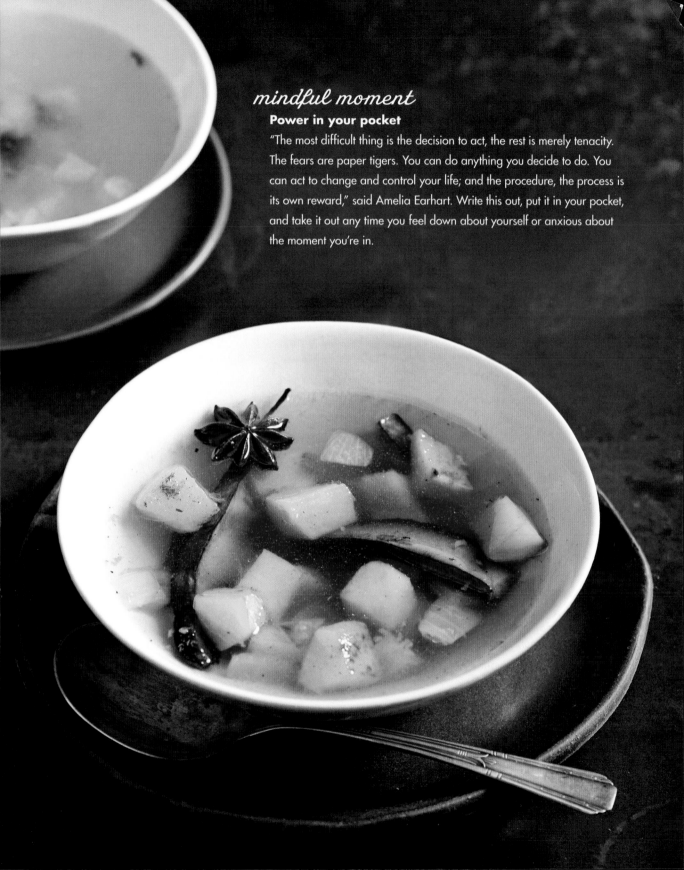

mindful moment
Power in your pocket

"The most difficult thing is the decision to act, the rest is merely tenacity. The fears are paper tigers. You can do anything you decide to do. You can act to change and control your life; and the procedure, the process is its own reward," said Amelia Earhart. Write this out, put it in your pocket, and take it out any time you feel down about yourself or anxious about the moment you're in.

horseradish has been used to treat a wide variety of ailments over the centuries, and nearly every part of the horseradish plant seems to have some medicinal value. Tea made from its root has been used as an expectorant, while tea brewed from its flowers can be used to fight the common cold. A poultice can also be made of its roots to externally treat joint discomfort. In addition, raw leaves of horseradish also fulfill a purpose as a natural analgesic, and when pressed against the forehead, can eliminate headache pain.

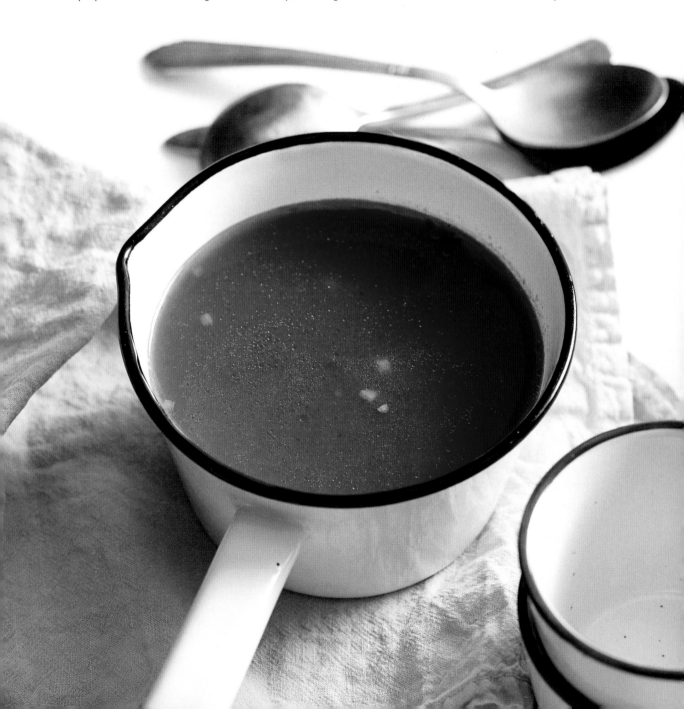

JALAPEÑO TOMATO BROTH

8   tomatoes or 2 cans (28 ounces each) no-salt-added crushed tomatoes (see note)

2   tablespoons olive oil

3   large cloves garlic, minced

1   jalapeño pepper, seeded and diced (use gloves if your skin is sensitive to hot peppers)

½   quart water

1   teaspoon sea salt

Ground black pepper, to taste

1   tablespoon grated fresh ginger

3   tablespoons prepared horseradish

Juice of 1 lime

1. Bring a large pot of water to a boil over high heat. Fill a mixing bowl with ice and water and set aside.

2. Core the stems of the tomatoes and slice a shallow "X" on the bottom of each one.

3. Gently place a few tomatoes at a time in the boiling water. Cook for 45 to 60 seconds, or until the skin begins to wrinkle. Using a slotted spoon, take the tomatoes out of the water and plunge them into the ice bath. Continue until all the tomatoes have been blanched.

4. Use your hands or a paring knife to remove the skins from the tomatoes.

5. Pulse the tomatoes in a food processor or pass them through a food mill until smooth.

6. In a large pot over medium heat, warm the oil. Cook the garlic and jalapeño pepper, stirring, for 3 to 5 minutes, or until fragrant.

7. Add the tomato puree, water, salt, black pepper, ginger, horseradish, and lime juice. Increase the heat to high and bring to a boil. Reduce the heat to medium and simmer for 30 minutes, stirring occasionally.

8. *Optional:* Pour the mixture through a fine colander lined with cheesecloth for a finer, clearer broth.

9. Serve hot or chilled.

■ WEIGHT LOSS
■ HEAL
■ DETOX

This is the perfect summertime soup, with a medley of flavors nearly as bright and bold as its red hue! I recommend using fresh tomatoes, in season from mid-May until October, to boost the flavor and impart the greatest amount of nutrients, the most important being our pal lycopene.

Note: Skip Steps 1 through 5 if using canned tomatoes. Or you can skip Steps 1 through 4 and just throw all the tomatoes into a food processor or blender if you don't mind skins and seeds!

SPIRULINA AND KALE

1   tablespoon olive oil

1   onion, sliced

2   cloves garlic, minced

2   tablespoons grated fresh ginger

½   teaspoon sea salt

1   teaspoon dried oregano

½   teaspoon ground red pepper

3   cups thinly sliced kale leaves (go with the Lacinato variety, if possible)

2½ quarts water

1   teaspoon spirulina powder

    Peel of 1 lemon, grated (about 2 teaspoons)

    Juice of 1 lemon

I talk about spirulina in Chapter 2, and here she is in all her deep-green algae glory. Spirulina can be tough to find, so feel free to substitute chopped-up nori seaweed, dried kelp, or wakame. Marine algae and seaweeds are a unique source of DHA omega-3 fatty acids, which are typically found in fatty fish, like salmon. These nutrient powerhouses are also high in iron and anti-inflammatory agents, which are fantastic for anyone recovering from or preparing for a big workout. More and more grocers carry these antioxidant-rich sea vegetables in dried form, but you can also just double up on kale if you can't find them.

1. In a large pot over medium heat, warm the oil. Add the onion and garlic and cook, stirring, for 7 to 10 minutes, or until the mixture is very soft. Stir in the ginger, salt, oregano, and red pepper and cook for 1 minute.

2. Add the kale and water. Increase the heat to high and bring to a boil. Reduce the heat to low and simmer, uncovered, for 1 hour, or until the liquid has reduced by about a quarter.

3. Turn off the heat and stir in the spirulina, lemon peel, and lemon juice.

4. Enjoy warm!

dear kale, inquiring minds want to know: Who are you, really? It's no wonder my mother-in-law is confused—every leaf has a different look, taste, and cooking temperament. The curly ones and spiky purple varieties (often called Red Russian) are my favorite for stews that like alone time at a slow simmer. The deep dark leaves will hold on to some of that raw green flavor if you slice them into thin ribbons and toss them into your soup at the last minute. Allow Lacinato to simmer a little longer, and the tough green flavor will soften a bit and contribute to a flavorful stock.

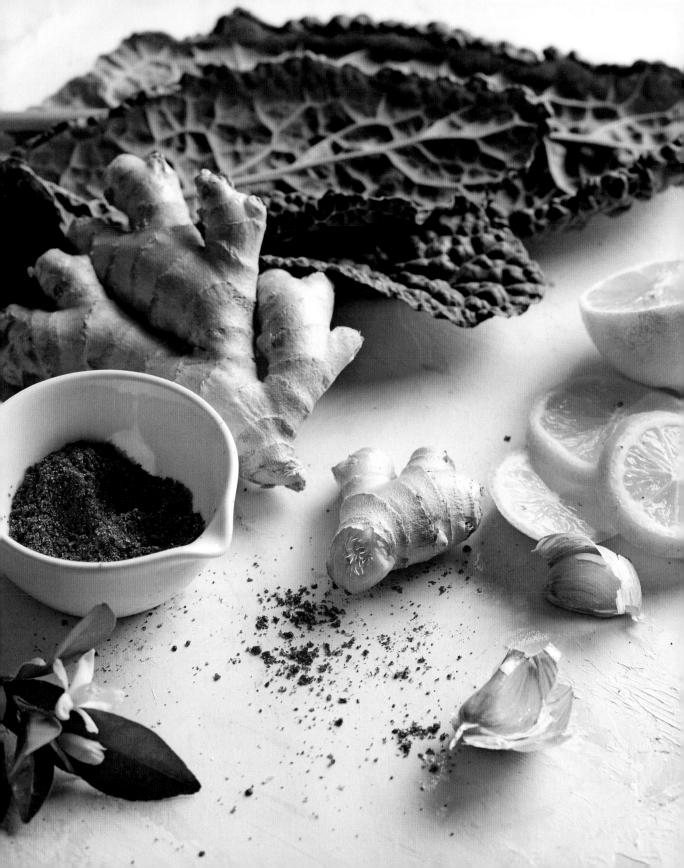

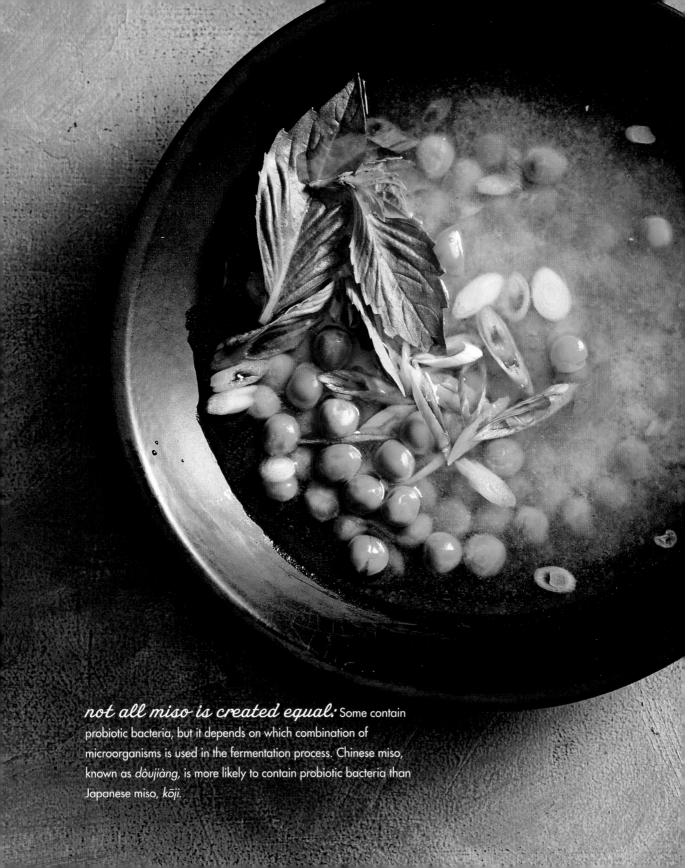

not all miso is created equal: Some contain probiotic bacteria, but it depends on which combination of microorganisms is used in the fermentation process. Chinese miso, known as *dòujiàng,* is more likely to contain probiotic bacteria than Japanese miso, *kōji.*

WHITE MISO *with* PEAS AND THAI BASIL

■ STRENGTHEN
■ HEAL
■ MOM AND BABY

1 tablespoon sesame oil or olive oil

4 scallions, sliced

1 clove garlic, chopped

1 quart water

4 tablespoons white miso

1½ cups fresh or frozen peas

1 cup Thai basil, torn

1. In a large pot over medium heat, warm the oil. Cook the scallions and garlic for 3 to 5 minutes, or until fragrant. Add the water. Increase the heat to high and bring to a boil. Reduce the heat to low so the water simmers as you prepare the miso.

2. In a small bowl, place the miso paste. Scoop out ½ cup of the hot water and pour over the miso. Stir with a whisk to dissolve until there are no lumps.

3. Add the peas to the pot. Increase the heat to medium and simmer for 10 minutes (if using frozen peas, reduce the time to 5 minutes).

4. Stir in the basil and miso paste right before serving.

5. Serve warm or chilled.

More umami here in this soothing white miso soup with fresh peas and peppery Thai basil. If you've never cooked with miso before, you're in for a treat. This staple in Chinese and Japanese cuisine is a paste made from fermented soybeans, salt, grains, and a fungus called *Aspergillus oryzae*. Fermented foods, like miso, are a good source of beneficial bacteria, protein, B vitamins, and dietary fiber.

mindful movement

Hug your world.

Wake up your body before you spoon by giving a "hug" to your world: Stretch your arms up toward the sky and open your heart to the environment around you. Repeat this movement throughout the day at any time you feel stressed or unsure of yourself. The physical act of making yourself longer and opening your chest toward the world will immediately shift your perception of the moment and give you deeper appreciation for simply being awake and open to the possibilities of the day. Stress is a temporary state, and you have the ability to be open to a fresher, calmer, more confident state at any time. You just have to reach out and receive it.

RED MISO *with* TURNIPS AND SESAME OIL

■ STRENGTHEN
■ MOM AND BABY

The longer fermentation period of a red miso means it has a deeper flavor that holds its own with heartier ingredients like black beans. Rich sesame oil warms the overall flavor, and turnips lighten up the texture with a bit of crunch.

1 tablespoon sesame oil or olive oil

1 small yellow onion, diced

1 clove garlic, minced

1 quart water

4 tablespoons red miso

½ cup dried black beans, soaked overnight and drained, or ⅓ can (5 ounces) low-sodium canned black beans, rinsed and drained

1 cup peeled and diced white turnips

1 tablespoon dried wakame

1. In a large pot over medium heat, warm the oil. Cook the onion and garlic, stirring, for 5 to 7 minutes, or until the mixture is soft and fragrant. Add the water. Increase the heat to high and bring to a boil. Reduce the heat to medium-low so the water simmers as you prepare the miso.

2. In a small bowl, place the miso paste. Scoop out ½ cup of the hot water and pour over the miso. Stir with a whisk to dissolve until there are no lumps.

3. Add the beans, turnips, and wakame to the pot. Increase the heat to medium and simmer for 15 minutes, or until the turnips and beans are soft.

4. Pour the miso mixture into the soup and stir to combine.

5. Serve warm.

WHAT'S THE DIFFERENCE BETWEEN WHITE, YELLOW, AND RED MISO?
There is a lot of conflicting information about the different types of miso, so let's clear things up.

- **WHITE MISO.** This miso is made from soybeans that have been fermented with a large percentage of rice. The actual resulting color can range from white to light beige, and the miso has a sweet taste. It's best used in condiments like mayo, salad dressings, or light sauces.

- **YELLOW MISO.** Yellow miso is usually made from soybeans that have been fermented with barley and sometimes a small percentage of rice. It can be yellow to light brown in color. This miso has a mild, earthy flavor and is better for general use in not only condiments but also soup, marinades, and glazes.

- **RED MISO.** This miso is also typically made from soybeans fermented with barley or other grains, but with a higher percentage of soybeans and/or a longer fermentation period. It can range in color from red to dark brown. The deep umami flavor of red miso can overwhelm mild dishes, but it is perfect for hearty soups, braises, and glazes.

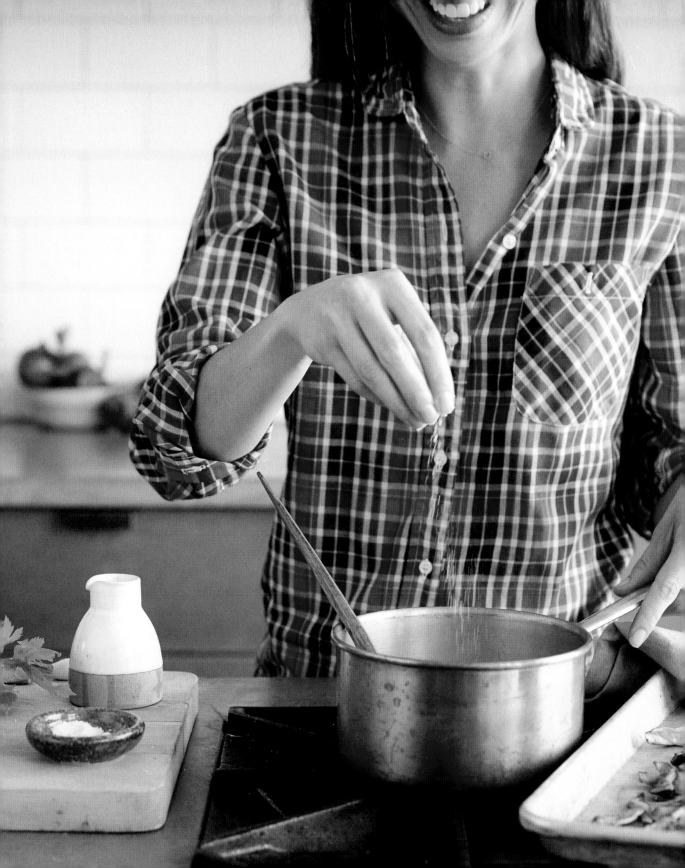

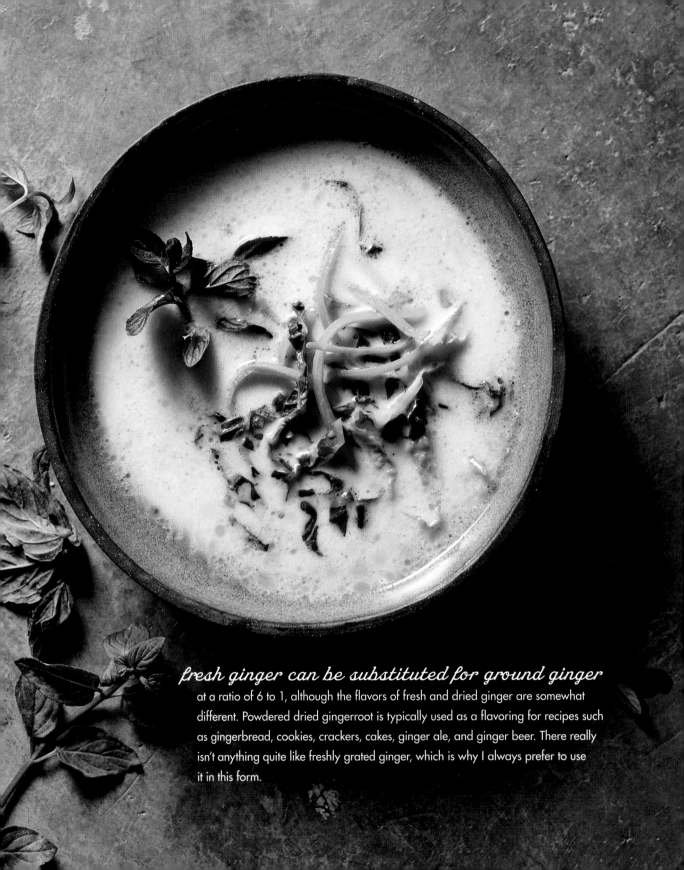

fresh ginger can be substituted for ground ginger at a ratio of 6 to 1, although the flavors of fresh and dried ginger are somewhat different. Powdered dried gingerroot is typically used as a flavoring for recipes such as gingerbread, cookies, crackers, cakes, ginger ale, and ginger beer. There really isn't anything quite like freshly grated ginger, which is why I always prefer to use it in this form.

GINGER BROTH *with* NAPA CABBAGE AND CARROTS

■HEAL
■DETOX
■ENERGIZE

This soup is bursting with flavor! Hardy carrots and crisp cabbage shine bright with color, delivering ample amounts of antioxidants and dietary fiber. Spicy ginger takes the lead, though, with a feisty kick of warmth that combats inflammation and calms your tummy.

2 tablespoons coconut oil

¼ jalapeño pepper, finely chopped (use gloves if your skin is sensitive to hot peppers)

2 scallions, thinly sliced

1 tablespoon grated ginger

2 cups thinly sliced napa cabbage

1 cup julienned or grated carrot

½ teaspoon sea salt plus more, to taste

1 quart water

1 can (15 ounces) coconut milk

Grated peel and juice of ½ orange

Ground black pepper, to taste

Mint leaves (optional)

1. In a large pot over medium heat, warm the oil. Cook the jalapeño pepper for 1 minute, or until soft. Add the scallions and ginger and cook for 30 seconds, or until fragrant.

2. Stir in the cabbage, carrots, and ½ teaspoon of the salt and cook, stirring occasionally, for 5 to 10 minutes, or until the cabbage and carrots have softened somewhat and the mixture is fragrant.

3. Add the water, coconut milk, orange peel, and orange juice, increase the heat to high, and bring to a boil. Reduce the heat to medium and simmer for 10 minutes, or until the carrots and cabbage are tender. Season with additional salt and the black pepper.

4. Serve warm or chilled with the mint, if using.

galangal is a fun substitute for ginger since it has a similar, albeit more delicate, somewhat floral flavor. Along with ginger, galangal belongs to the *Zingiberaceae* family, which includes turmeric and cardamom. Galangal is in the homemade green curry paste on page 158, but you can substitute it for ginger in any of the recipes.

CLASSIC FILIPINO SINIGANG

2   tablespoons olive oil

1   small yellow onion, diced

1   clove garlic, minced

1   cup chopped eggplant

1   teaspoon tamarind paste

1½ quarts water

1½ teaspoons sea salt plus more, to taste

1   small white potato, diced

1   cup halved green beans, ends removed

1   tomato, diced

    Ground black pepper, to taste

1   calamansi or small lime, sliced into wedges

1. In a large pot over medium heat, warm the oil. Cook the onion, garlic, and eggplant, stirring, for 5 to 10 minutes, or until the mixture is soft.

2. Stir in the tamarind paste, water, and the 1½ teaspoons salt. Increase the heat to medium-high and bring to a simmer. Add the potato and cook for 15 minutes, or until the potato is tender.

3. Add the green beans and tomato and simmer for 5 minutes, or until the green beans are al dente. Season with additional salt and the pepper.

4. Serve hot with the calamansi or lime wedges.

Sinigang is a Filipino stew characterized by its sour and savory taste. Its hearty, happy flavor comes from the tartness of tamarind paste, the bright crunch of crisp green beans, the earthy notes of eggplant, and a zesty splash of calamansi (or lime) juice at the end. This stew is often made with a pork hock or a flaky white fish or a chicken foot or basically any other meat you may have that would benefit from a slow simmer. My grandmother usually made it with beef shank, and I slurped down bowl after steaming-hot bowl, watching the fatty meat create pools of oil on the surface. As an adult, when I longed for this stew, it was the tangy-tart broth that I remembered, and not so much the fatty meats. This plant-based version is much lighter and fresher than the broth I had as a child, but it is every bit as fortifying.

calamansi is like a cross between a mandarin and a lime, with a sweet peel and sour pulp/juice. It's actually a hybrid between a member of the citrus family and the kumquat, and it is commonly used as a condiment in Filipino dishes.

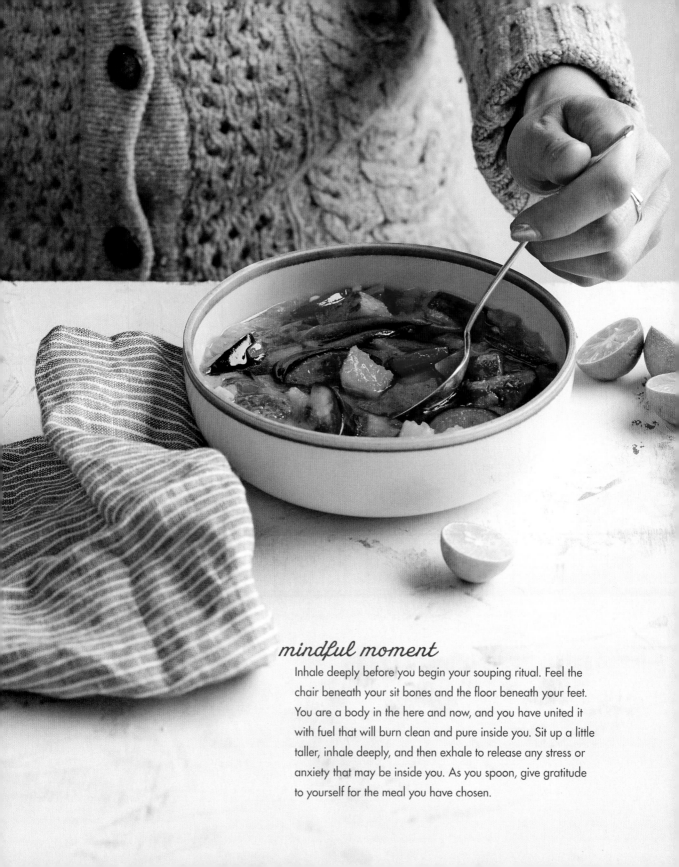

mindful moment

Inhale deeply before you begin your souping ritual. Feel the
chair beneath your sit bones and the floor beneath your feet.
You are a body in the here and now, and you have united it
with fuel that will burn clean and pure inside you. Sit up a little
taller, inhale deeply, and then exhale to release any stress or
anxiety that may be inside you. As you spoon, give gratitude
to yourself for the meal you have chosen.

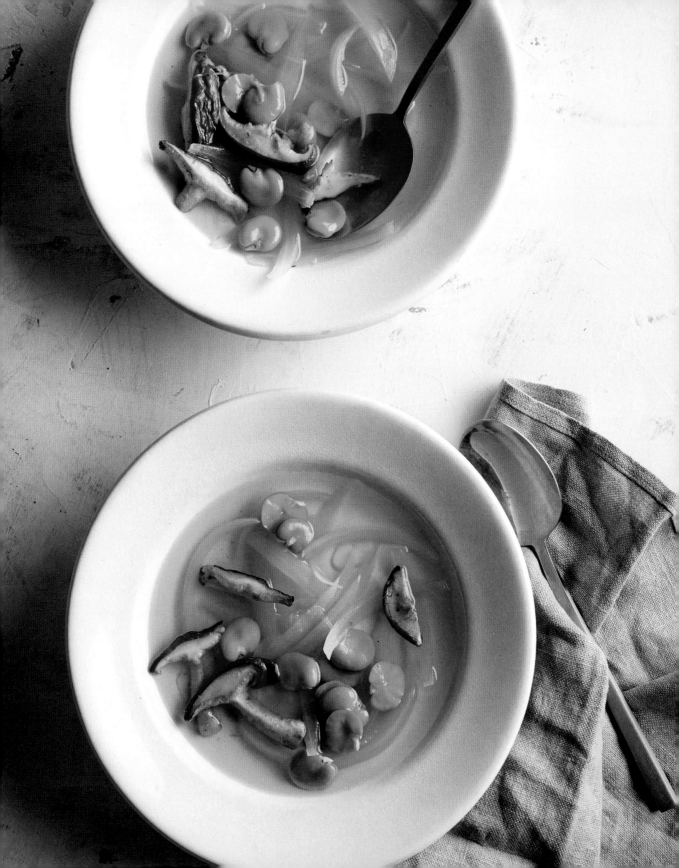

FAVAS *and* MORELS IN MUSHROOM BROTH

2–3 ounces dried mushrooms (any variety)

½ small onion, thinly sliced

2 cloves garlic, thinly sliced

1 tablespoon thinly sliced fresh ginger

1 tablespoon chopped fresh marjoram or oregano

2 cups mushroom stems (any variety), wrapped in cheesecloth

2½ quarts water

1 cup morels or shiitake mushrooms, sliced

1 cup fresh fava beans or frozen fava or lima beans

½ teaspoon sea salt

Juice of ½ lemon

1. In a large pot over high heat, bring the dried mushrooms, onion, garlic, ginger, marjoram or oregano, mushroom stems, and water to a boil. Reduce the heat to medium-low and simmer for 25 minutes, or until the mushroom stems are very soft. Turn off the heat. Remove the mushroom stem parcel and discard.

2. Add the morels or shiitakes, beans, and salt, cover, and allow the carry-over heat to cook the mixture for 8 minutes, or until cooked through. Add the lemon juice.

3. Enjoy this soup warm, and try to catch a morel or fava bean in every spoonful for the best flavor experience.

PREPARING FRESH FAVA BEANS

Preparing fresh fava beans is a two-step process. (1) Remove the beans from the tough outer pod and discard the pod. (2) Remove the bright green beans from their opaque outer casings (I usually break a little hole in the outer casing and then squeeze the bean out). The fresh buttery flavor of these seasonal beans is totally worth the extra effort.

■ WEIGHT LOSS
■ STRENGTHEN

I think of favas and morels as spring's sexier, more mysterious progeny. Where asparagus and chives cheerfully present themselves alert and ready to eat straight from the market stand, favas and morels take a little more effort to find and enjoy. Everything else about this soup is incredibly quick and easy.

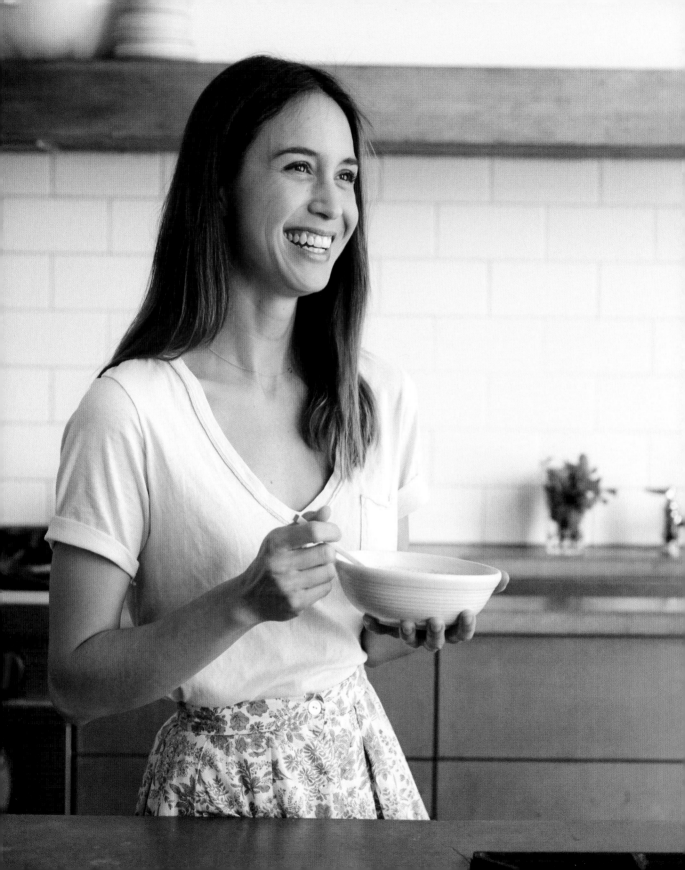

ENDNOTES

CHAPTER 1

1 "Profiling Food Consumption in America," *USDA Office of Communications Agriculture Fact Book, 2001–2002* (Washington, DC: US Government Printing Office, 2003), 13–19.

2 Tom Philpott, "The American Diet in One Chart, with Lots of Fats and Sugars," Grist.org, April 6, 2011, grist.org/industrial-agriculture/2011-04-05 -american-diet-one-chart-lots-of-fats-sugars/.

3 "FastStats: Obesity and Overweight," Centers for Disease Control and Prevention, last modified February 25, 2016, cdc.gov/nchs/fastats/obesity-overweight.htm.

4 "FastStats: Leading Causes of Death," Centers for Disease Control and Prevention, last modified February 25, 2016, cdc.gov/nchs/fastats/leading-causes-of -death.htm.

5 "The Nutrition Source: Vegetables and Fruit," Harvard T. H. Chan School of Public Health, accessed March 7, 2016, hsph.harvard.edu/nutritionsource /what-should-you-eat/vegetables-and-fruits; Frank B. Hu, "Plant-Based Foods and Prevention of Cardiovascular Disease: An Overview," *American Journal of Clinical Nutrition* 78, no. S3 (September 2003): 544S–51S.

6 Latetia V. Moore and Frances E. Thompson, "Adults Meeting Fruit and Vegetable Intake Recommendations— United States, 2013," *Morbidity and Mortality Weekly Report* 64, no. 26 (July 10, 2015): 709–13.

7 Jennifer M. Poti et al., "Is the Degree of Food Processing and Convenience Linked with the Nutritional Quality of Foods Purchased by US Households?" *American Journal of Clinical Nutrition* 101, no. 6 (May 5, 2014): 1251–62.

8 Philpott, "American Diet in One Chart."

9 Ann Gibbons, "The Evolution of Diet," *National Geographic*, accessed February 24, 2016, nationalgeographic.com/foodfeatures/evolution-of-diet/.

10 Ibid.

11 Dan Buettner, "The Island Where People Forget to Die," *New York Times Magazine*, October 24, 2012, nytimes.com/2012/10/28/magazine/the-island-where -people-forget-to-die.html?_r=0.

12 Dan Pardi, "Does Protein Restriction and Fasting Slow the Aging Process? Better Aging Part 3," *Dan's Plan* (blog), December 9, 2015, blog.dansplan.com /does-protein-restriction-and-fasting-slow-the-aging -process-better-aging-part-3/.

13 J. B. Johnson, D. R. Laub, and S. John, "The Effect on Health of Alternate Day Calorie Restriction: Eating Less and More Than Needed on Alternate Days Prolongs Life," *Medical Hypotheses* 67, no. 2 (2006): 209–11; Eliza Barclay, "Eating to Break 100: Longevity Tips from the Blue Zones," *NPR The Salt*, April 11, 2015, npr.org/sections/thesalt/2015/04/11 /398325030/eating-to-break-100-longevity-diet-tips- from-the-blue-zones.

14 "Product Gallery," Water Footprint Network, accessed March 7, 2016, waterfootprint.org/en /resources/interactive-tools/product-gallery.

15 Peter Scarborough et al., "Dietary Greenhouse Gas Emissions of Meat-Eaters, Fish-Eaters, Vegetarians and Vegans in the UK," *Climatic Change* 125, no. 2 (July 2014): 179–92.

16 R. J. Davidson et al., "Alterations in Brain and Immune Function Produced by Mindfulness Meditation," *Psychosomatic Medicine* 65, no. 4 (July–August 2003): 564–70.

17 M. E. Clegg et al., "Soups Increase Satiety through Delayed Gastric Emptying Yet Increased Glycaemic Response," *European Journal of Clinical Nutrition* 67, no. 1 (January 2013): 8–11.

18 Michaeleen Doucleff, "Got Gas? It Could Mean You've Got Healthy Gut Microbes," *NPR The Salt*, April 28, 2014, npr.org/sections/thesalt/2014/04/28 /306544406/got-gas-it-could-mean-you-ve-got- healthy-gut-microbes.

CHAPTER 2

1   L. V. Moore and F. E. Thompson, "Adults Meeting Fruit and Vegetable Intake Recommendations—United States, 2013," *Morbidity and Mortality Weekly Report* 64, no. 26 (July 10, 2015): 709–13.

2   "FastStats: Obesity and Overweight," Centers for Disease Control and Prevention, last modified February 25, 2016, cdc.gov/nchs/fastats/obesity-overweight.htm.

3   T. T. Fung and F. B. Hu, "Plant-Based Diets: What Should Be on the Plate?" *American Journal of Clinical Nutrition* 78, no. 3 (September 2003): 357–58.

4   Lynne Olver, "Why Do We Call It Soup?" Food Timeline, accessed February 24, 2016, foodtimeline.org/foodsoups.html#soupword.

5   Kaye Spector, "Raw Veggies Pack a Punch, But Cooking Can Unlock Key Benefits," Cleveland.com, August 3, 2010, cleveland.com/healthfit/index.ssf/2010/08/raw_veggies_can_pack_a_punch_b.html.

6   Blaine Friedlander, "Italian Chefs Knew It All Along: Cooking Plump Red Tomatoes Boosts Disease-Fighting, Nutritional Power, Cornell Researchers Say," *Cornell Chronicle*, April 19, 2002, news.cornell.edu/stories/2002/04/cooking-tomatoes-boosts-disease-fighting-power.

7   "Beta-Carotene," WebMD, accessed February 24, 2016, www.webmd.com/vitamins-supplements/ingredientmono-999-beta-carotene.aspx?active ingredientid=999&activeingredientname=beta-carotene.

8   Cristiana Miglio et al., "Effects of Different Cooking Methods on Nutritional and Physicochemical Characteristics of Selected Vegetables," *Journal of Agricultural and Food Chemistry* 56, no. 1 (January 2008): 139–47.

9   S. T. Talcott, L. R. Howard, and C. H. Brenes, "Antioxidant Changes and Sensory Properties of Carrot Puree Processed with and without Periderm Tissue," *Journal of Agricultural and Food Chemistry* 48, no. 4 (April 2000): 1315–21.

10 Zahid Naeem, "Vitamin D Deficiency—An Ignored Epidemic," *International Journal of Health Sciences* 4, no. 1 (January 2010): v–vi.

11 "The Nutrition Source: Fiber," Harvard T. H. Chan School of Public Health, accessed February 24, 2016, hsph.harvard.edu/nutritionsource/carbohydrates/fiber/.

12 Diane E. Threapleton et al., "Dietary Fibre Intake and Risk of Cardiovascular Disease: Systematic Review and Meta-Analysis," *BMJ* 347 (December 19, 2003): f6879.

ACKNOWLEDGMENTS

A WOMAN WALKS ARM-IN-ARM with her crew, and here's mine. Mama! You glow so brightly that my world has always been illuminated. I see beauty and opportunity and hope when I open my eyes each morning, and I have you to thank for this. You are my guide and my inspiration, and I'm so grateful to know your spirit begot mine. Papa! I have a greater capacity for self-love and independence because I have seen these traits evolve in you, my father. I am incredibly fortunate to have been raised by a man who shows strength through empathy and compassion. Courtney, dear younger sister, I look up to you now. Thank you for pointing out fragments and my overuse of the word *amazing*. Thank you for being my older sister when I need one. Brian, there is so much of you and me in the story of Splendid Spoon. Thank you for your friendship, thank you for allowing our love to evolve, thank you for being a wonderful dad to our two boys. Grover and Caleb: my mountain and my sun. Some day you will read this and know that I was reborn along with you both. I am forever grateful to you for showing me strength and vulnerability, and the need for both. Diana, Diana, Diana. You were destined to become entwined in my life the day you showed up with Pants and became my surprise third roommate. I will always be in debt to you for your endless well of support and love, and I haven't even touched on the countless hours of work you put into making this book happen. Emma, you have been a consistent source

of confidence, relief, and encouragement throughout this very fast-paced project. Thank you for being who you are: obsessed with detail; committed to timelines; in love with food; and, above all, a compassionate friend, wife, and mother. There would be no recipes, no cookbook, without you. Thanks Mitchell and Ada for sharing this special woman with me for this project. I'm still amazed by the unique beauty and strength that my Spoon Crew shares with me every day, and I'm grateful that each of you saw what I saw when there was very little to be seen. Leah, you embody the spirit and voice of Splendid Spoon because it is true to who you are. Thank you for your smarts, your sense of humor, and your care. Sathish, you are my brother from another mother. I am so grateful for our partnership. I hope I continue to inspire you in the same way that you motivate me. Rene, you may not have worked directly on this book, but your heart is in every page. I thank the sun for casting a beam of light on you just as our paths crossed. Thank you Jane von Mehren for *really* kicking my butt into action to write this first book. I hope this is just the beginning. Marisa Vigilante! You are so supportive it hurts. Thank you for taking a chance on me. Thank you for pushing me to be clearer, sharper, better. I hope this is just the beginning for you and me, too. Thank you Tara Donne for taking soup for payment for way too long. Your eye is uncanny, and I'm so fortunate to have your images grace these pages. Thank you Isabelle Hughes for making me feel at home throughout every step of this process . . . and for honoring my midnight, or sometimes 4 a.m., deadlines! Thank you, Team Rodale: Gail Gonzales, Jennifer Levesque, Melissa Miceli, Sindy Berner, Chris Gaugler, and Hope Clarke. Thank you to Martha Bernabe, Hadas Smirnoff, and Prop Haus for making the pages of this book come alive with your careful eye for detail and beauty. Colleen Rafferty—girl, you started this. Big thanks to my partners in life and business for believing in me. If you're listed here, you have invested in me in some big way, whether it be smart advice, pro-bono work with the Spoon Crew, an open-door policy at your home, capital, or most important of all, being a true friend: Kelsey Kyro, Lani Free, Jason Lepes, Scott Crawford, Ali Pugliese, Anthony Robustelli, Greg Stefano, Ami Kealoha, Amy and Govindasami Naadimuthu, Alexis Ohanian, Chris and Emily Tomson, Tom and Cevrem Campbell, Nick and Tessa Mencia, Elisabeth and Tyler Pulvermann, Carl Forsberg, Helen White, Jim White, Alex Gorman, Rebecca Connolly, DJ Haley, Dan Glickberg, Dan Pardi, Allison Monti, Karin Weidenmueller, Chivas deVinck, Sarah Watson, Karen Freer, Murf Meyer, my Centeno clan, my MacDonald clan, my Arcellana clan, Lexi Green, Noah Rosenberg, Liz Fulton, Fane Googins, Zach Haigney, Anne Reilly, Monique Hypes, Billy Clark, Michael Krueger, and Nick Dziekonski. I'm so grateful to all of you!

INDEX